THE PRAYER OF SILENCE

A Complete Course in Spiritual Transformation

Bruce Fraser MacDonald, PhD

Author of *THE THOMAS BOOK:*
Near Death, a Quest and a New Gospel by the Twin Brother of Jesus
(Eloquent Books, 2010)

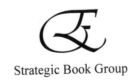

Strategic Book Group

Strategic Book Group
P.O. Box 333
Durham CT 06422
www.StrategicBookClub.com

ISBN: 978-1-60911-574-6

Book Design: Stacie Tingen

Dedicated to the Source of all inspiration
Without whose Breath,
Neither this book, nor this life,
Would have been.

Contents

Acknowledgements

There are so many people I would like to thank because you have contributed to my life.

First I thank my immediate family – Olive, David and Rachel – and later Dana and Gulliver who joined the adventure. My life and my search have been difficult. You have shared that life and we have had difficult times as well as good times together. I hope you have benefited from it all. Thank you, Olive, for reading over the manuscript and making suggestions and corrections, and especially for being with me all those years, even when the going was tough. You cannot know how much that has meant to me.

I also thank the family into which I was born – Dad and Mom (Peter and Edna), Marilyn, Eric and Ian. Ours has been an "interesting life." Thanks for sharing those years.

Thank you to Dr. William Wynn, psychologist and friend, for inviting me to speak to your classes and for asking the difficult questions, so that I had to put my experiences into a form which others could understand. Thank you also to my colleague and friend at Luther College, Dr. Paul Antrobus, another psychologist, for all the discussions we shared of alternative ways of seeing things. Thank you Dami Egbeyemi, for showing me more of how my brain works with your computer and Brain State Technologies®.

I thank the Sunday Morning Study Group at Wesley United Church in Regina, Saskatchewan, Canada, for providing a place where ideas of all sorts could be discussed freely.

And I thank the many members of the meditation classes and groups I have led over the years at Whitmore Park United Church, the University of Regina and a variety of community groups. I learned so much from you all.

To contact the author please write to: TheThomasBook@gmail.com

Author's website: www.ThomasTwin.com

Introduction

At first I could not see any relationship between my Near Death Experience and meditation, or between these two and the teachings of Jesus. I knew there was something connecting them, because I kept coming back to all three whenever I thought of spiritual growth and transformation or the many spiritual experiences I had in those years of searching.

My experiences were certainly not of the usual type. After the Near Death Experience (NDE) in 1966, I was able to re-activate my dead body through a particular aspect of consciousness I discovered while "on the other side." In the early 1980s, I was able to enter in meditation into an intimate relationship with Jesus, and through that was able to write a Gospel, *The Thomas Book: Near Death, a Quest and a New Gospel by the Twin Brother of Jesus* (Eloquent Books, 2010). It was while writing that book that I was introduced to "the Prayer of Silence." This Prayer of Silence turned out to be not just one prayer, but a whole integrated approach to spiritual growth and comprehensive healing. In 1991 I was able to use the skills, learned in practicing the Prayer of Silence, to recover from a severe case of viral encephalitis which wiped out most of my memory. But the relationship between all of these was certainly not obvious for a long time. Nor was it easy to teach what I had experienced or to put all of this in an order which would make sense to others.

During the Near Death Experience, I discovered an aspect of my consciousness which could act independently of the body and could access areas of awareness that I knew nothing about before that experience. I called this aspect of my consciousness, "the Watcher," because that title seemed to fit how I felt during the NDE. I watched what was going on. But I also participated actively in the death of the body and the transition to "the other side." At the end of the NDE, it was the Watcher which made it possible for me to return to life when Jesus gave me the choice whether to stay over there or to return to a badly smashed up body. Later, the Watcher became the agent through which I was able to find healing for my body and all other aspects of my life.

I sensed that all of this was related to meditation and to Jesus' teachings as recorded in the New Testament. But I wondered how I could clarify my intuition that this was the case. And how could I teach this new knowledge to people raised in the traditional values and ideas of Christianity, or even to people who had no connection with the church? It seemed to me that this new awareness would be of benefit, not just to church members, but to everyone, from all backgrounds, but I knew I could not leave out Jesus' teachings, because they made unified sense of all of my experience.

I was especially interested in solving the problem of whether I could teach to other people, something which had taken me a Near Death Experience and many years of inner work, guided from within by Jesus and other spiritual teachers. Would it bring them the same benefit it had brought me? I knew I had to explore that.

In my own life, it made a tremendous difference, and in counselling others, it helped to resolve difficulties of long standing – sometimes helping with problems from which people had suffered for years, things that had not responded to psychiatric and other medical treatment. But as the years went by, and I entered deeper into the levels of consciousness which were opened by meditation, and as I led meditation groups and taught the healing benefits of the Prayer of Silence, I knew I had to put all of this into writing. However difficult it was to organize and express, I knew that others needed to hear what I had done and what they could do with the Prayer of Silence.

And they kept asking, "When are you going to write all this down? Let me know so I can get a copy, because it must not be allowed to just disappear when you are gone."

I discovered that I could introduce people to exercises which almost duplicated in meditation, the Watcher awareness I had experienced in the NDE. Others could tap into the healing benefits of that level of awareness very quickly. And I also discovered that all of what I had learned was prefigured in the New Testament teachings of Jesus. In fact, exploring his teachings helped to clarify many of the theoretical aspects of the Prayer of Silence.

In Jesus' parables and other sayings, I found the clues I needed to teach others the spiritual framework within which this Prayer of Silence made sense. I even began to wonder if this Prayer of Silence was somehow implied in or assumed as a background for many of the things people recorded that Jesus said. There seemed to have been some kind of spiritual practice involved in Jesus' teachings, but that spiritual practice has been lost because it was not recorded by his disciples.

Exploring all of this, I could also understand where I had gone in death and also where we go in meditation, because it is essentially the same place. When we die and when we meditate we enter into the same spiritual realms.

Once I discovered that I could teach others to enter into the Watcher consciousness, and to benefit from the healing and creative potential of the Prayer of Silence, it was then time to write this book, in stages, to guide others into the deep, inner peace, assurance and creativity which come from the regular practice of the Prayer of Silence. I knew that I could teach others in small group settings. Would it be possible to put all of this into a book and organize it in a way that people could follow?

Much of this material was originally presented to small groups, and I have tried to maintain the oral style of the original. I address you as a person, not as a distant theoretical idea. I hope I have given you, the reader, a sense of being intimately involved in all that I write here. I hope you feel you can enter into the ideas and exercises in a personal way and that you feel personally involved in what I have presented here. That is my aim, because this experience of entering into the Prayer of Silence is very personal. It will change who you are, forever. And that change will be tremendously positive as you come to know the deepest feelings and longings of the heart, and how you can grow and be transformed in your search for a close relationship with others and with God.

Finally, it all came together after years of practice, searching and teaching others. In the pages that follow, you can learn to enter into the Silence of God where our true Being lies. As Jesus said so often, "The Kingdom of God is within you." These pages will help you to enter into that Kingdom and become aware of your oneness with the Divine Source of your Being.

Chapter One

The Prayer of Silence: An Overview

In some ways, I wish this Prayer of Silence was different, that I could have a snappy way of introducing the Silence, something that would reach out and grab you and draw you into the centre of the subject. The problem is, that would be an aim very different from the experience of this Prayer. The snappy opening would reflect a world of power and instant effect, something more akin to ego gratification and our noisy world of pull, push, shove, grab, hit, defend, judge.

The Prayer of Silence is different: you come to it quietly and find it in stillness. The centre of this Prayer is the simple act of consciously being still and silent. We move our attention from the outer world, where we have to live, to the inner world, where we can learn to live more fully.

Strange as it may seem, what sets this Prayer apart from other methods of meditation and prayer, is that the Prayer of Silence is based on a different perception of death, a perception which arose in the first place when I had a profound Near Death Experience in 1966, but which you will be able to accomplish through daily practice. You will be taught how to achieve the perspective achieved in death, so that you can rise to a new life over and over.

There is something very special about this "death." Seeing from its perspective, you will be able to learn a great deal about yourself as a spiritual being -- things which cannot be perceived when you look only from the view of a mortal creature looking for meaning in a seemingly mortal existence. Here, you will know yourself to be immortal every time you enter the Silence, and you will be transformed by that knowledge.

In the exercises and theoretical discussion in this book, you will be introduced to an aspect of your consciousness which you use every day without being aware of its significance. I call this "the Watcher," named after the being seen by King Nebuchadnezzar in his dream in the Book of Daniel in the Bible. The King said to Daniel, "I saw in the visions of my head while on my bed, and there was a watcher, a holy one, coming down from Heaven" (Dan 4:13). It is time to become aware of this Watcher, of the divine centre of your being, the holy one who comes from the Kingdom of Heaven which is within you.

Slowly, by following the exercises in this book, you will be able to put the negative aspects of the ego aside. You will let go of all the attachments of fear, anger, revenge, hatred and other selfish, violent things, and you will cultivate the Divine Ego, the awareness of the Divine Presence around and within you. Then, from the One Source, deep within you, love and light and joy and peace will begin to shine.

In these pages, we go step by step through a radically different way of bringing about healing of our bodies, relationships and societies. After a time of coming regularly into the Silence of the Self and the Silence of God, we find that our consciousness has itself been totally transformed.

Just reading the book will change your whole orientation in life. Practicing the exercises as well will lead you to an understanding of a spiritual depth within you which you may not have known you had.

As you go through the book, and especially in the last chapter, you will find a growing sense of oneness with the Divine Mystery at the heart of your being. It is this experience of Divine Union which the great spiritual masters of every culture have spoken about, what St. Paul refers to when he writes to the Galatians to tell them he will continue to teach them "until Christ is formed in you" (Gal 4:19). The Christ is something which grows within you. This divine oneness is within your reach.

You do not have to be holy or special to achieve spiritual fulfilment – the Watcher aspect of your being is always within you, waiting to be activated, no matter what your personal or moral condition right now. It might even help if you do have at least some darkness to overcome. Usually, the people who think they have everything right in their lives, do not bother to search for what we are seeking, and so they miss out on the most valuable things in life. Be willing to look at the darkness within you and you will find a much greater light.

I have gone into the depths of great darkness and great suffering in myself and have found a meaning which is not destroyed by that darkness. I smashed up my body so severely in an industrial accident when I was a young man that I died. The insights which were the basis of this Prayer of Silence came in a profound Near Death Experience following that accident. I was given a choice to stay "over there" or return. I decided to return. When I came back, it took seven months merely to be able to get out of the hospital on crutches and braces, and many years after that before I finally realized how this Prayer of Silence could transform my life. It was then that the real healing began.

Later, in the middle of my career as a university professor, I had viral encephalitis -- inflammation of the lining of the brain -- which destroyed career, family, memory and everything that I was. As my daughter said, "One day my Dad was there, then the next he was gone and someone else was left." I couldn't recognize friends or sign my name or copy numbers. However, by the time I had this severe brain damage, I had been practicing and teaching the Prayer of Silence for many years and was able to use it to put my memory, my brain and my life back together. In the process of healing my brain and my body, I found a peace, love and joy which go far deeper than any physical healing possibly could.

So do not worry if you are in the middle of painful experiences of the body or emotions or relationships. That is where you start. That is where you enter the Silence. And from there you move to find a spiritual centre of peace within you and a spiritual power of healing surrounding you, which will transform your life.

In this book, I am sharing something that works. I have used it in the darkest experiences of suffering and illness and pain -- in areas where the medical experts told me there was nothing that could be done to help me. I know from personal experience that it works. It is not just positive or happy ideas, however helpful those can be. It works when you do not even have the energy to generate happy thoughts -- in all the grungy and dark areas of life which we try to hide even from ourselves. It works where positive thoughts and intentions, where religious or scientific beliefs, where pills and drugs and all conventional aids fail us.

I am not the only one who has benefited. It has worked for many people I have counselled through severe trauma. It has worked for church and university groups to whom I have taught some of what is included here. It has worked for people who have read a shorter version of this book in manuscript form and have found it extremely helpful in putting their lives back together after tragedy, injury, accident or loss.

My claims, then, come from my own experience and from the experience of others I have been privileged to help. In these pages is a distillation of the ideas, exercises, experiences and stories which have proved themselves effective in transforming the lives of many people. It can transform your life as well.

[I must caution that what is included here is not intended to replace professional medical or psychiatric treatment. I have benefited from the skill of doctors and nurses and the appropriate drugs when I needed them, and I am very thankful to them for their skill, caring and effectiveness. If you have medical or psychiatric problems, see a doctor. The methods described here are designed for life-long transformation, not short-term treatment of medical problems. They can, however, help to increase the effectiveness of any medical treatment, because they will often help to resolve the underlying personal problems which gave rise to the illness in the first place.]

Chapter Two

Daily Silence – The Beginning

I learned the initial stages of the Prayer of Silence while I was writing *The Thomas Book*. In fact, some of the instructions for this form of meditation and the philosophy behind it were written right into that book. I quote the following paragraphs because they summarize, more clearly than I could, how to begin the Prayer of Silence. The words are from the perspective of Judas Thomas, one of Jesus' disciples, the one through whom *The Thomas Book* was partly written, and they tell how the disciples first learned to pray the interior prayer of Jesus:

> *Those first few days I seemed to learn little, but a great peace grew steadily over me. It was the prayer he instructed us in which brought this peace. Every morning and evening we sat silently for a time, letting the cares of the world drain from us and being filled in imagination with the light of the Father.*
>
> *When we did this meditation on fine mornings, outside, while we faced the rising sun, we began to feel all the light and life of the world rise up within us.*
>
> *In the evening, we let the day die within us, that we might not be bound by it, but might be born anew each evening and morning.*
>
> *This was the centre of our life, this prayer, this meditation. And I began to see those inner doors open, which I had closed out of fear or hatred. Gradually, as my eyes turned inward, I began to see as I had never seen.*
>
> *'You will indeed see and hear and speak things which have been hidden from humanity since the founding of the earth,' he told us one morning as we sat on a grassy slope.*

'You see with your eyes like all people, but you do not see.
What can the eyes show you or the ears tell you? They can tell
you of the surfaces of things. But I will lead you into a deeper
way. You will see into the things themselves.'

'And with your hands and eyes you know your body, but
I will show you a knowledge of your body and your heart and
mind and Spirit. You will see your mind and know your Spirit
and understand the longings and desires of the heart.'

'Do you not already feel within you the peace which leads
to understanding? You will be able to move in that peace to
know the Father as I know the Father.'

(From the words of Judas Thomas, *The Thomas Book*, p. 112-113)

Meditation Exercise: Daily review and prayer

The nice thing about this passage is that it gives you all the instructions you need to begin meditation. This is the first exercise in the book. Twice a day is all that is required. In the evening you sit quietly and comfortably, close your eyes and review the events of the day. When you have finished your review, imagine the conflicts from your day flowing from you like warm water. Then imagine you are surrounding yourself with light and sit for a time in that light, sensing that God is present with you. Spend some time in the silence and the light. When you are ready, thank God for whatever you have received and go to sleep when you are ready.

In the morning you do the same. Sit or lie comfortably and silently, with eyes closed. Review anything from the night before. Then, once you have noted anything you want to note, imagine the events of the night flowing from you. Imagine the day before you, with any special concerns. Ask for God's guidance during the day. Then visualize the light of God surrounding you and invite God to be present with you. Spend some time in the silence and the light. Then, when you are ready, thank God for anything you have received, allow the night to slip from you and prepare for the day.

You might even want to try meditating outside sometimes while the sun is rising. It is a beautiful and peaceful time of day, with the birds singing and the air still and crisp, before the bustle of the day begins. The evening is often a lovely time for meditation outside. Just as the sun is slipping below the horizon, the whole world seems to enter into rest, the birds chirp in the trees as they settle for the night and the world enters into peace. At that time, there is a special stillness in the air which can become part of you as well. You will begin in this way to enter into the rhythm of nature as the world wakes and as the world sleeps.

There is nothing you have to achieve here. You are just being invited into the silence and the peace of God and are allowing the things of the day or the night to slip from you for a while.

You are also learning some very important lessons. What you imagine in your mind actually begins to happen. When you imagine the problems of the world slipping from you, you are actually giving your inner being permission to let go of the things that bother you and you are preparing the inner conditions which will result in the outer changes you want to see. When you imagine the light of God around you, you are actually permitting God to enter into your personal space. When you enter into inner peace, you will begin to find where God lives in your life. The Kingdom of God is within you, as Jesus said. In this meditation you are finally discovering where you can find God.

There is a passage from the Psalms which is often quoted in relation to prayer and meditation: "Be still and know that I am God." (Ps 46:10) This is the motto of the Prayer of Silence. We begin with the stillness of the simple morning and evening meditation, and go on from there to explore many of the aspects of what Jesus called "The Kingdom of God," which he said is in us all. "In my Father's house are many mansions," he said. As you spend more time in the Silence, you begin to discover a great deal about how God is manifest within you, the temple of God.

One thing that cannot be done in a book is to anticipate the passage of time. I cannot assume that you will do the above exercise for a few days before going on to the next. However, I can say that it is not necessary to hurry from one exercise to the next, or to try to finish the whole book and all its exercises in a short time. What is included here can take your whole life to complete. Some people will want to read through the whole book to get a sense of the total shape of its contents, and some may want to take one step at a time. In either case, do not feel like you have to hurry on to the next exercise. You may want to savour each step before moving on to the next.

However, when you are ready, or even to add to the daily exercise outlined above, there are two things I would like to add to the simple description of the Prayer of Silence from *The Thomas Book*. One is a form of progressive relaxation which will help you to focus on what you want to achieve in meditation. The other is a way of correcting any errors you find in your life.

***

Meditation Exercise: Progressive relaxation

You will use this progressive relaxation many times in your spiritual life and in the meditation exercises in this book. It is a foundational exercise, so it would be good for you to spend some time perfecting it, and remembering the stages through which you achieve the desired relaxed awareness which is its aim.

It would be possible to record this exercise on a CD and listen to it every time you do your meditation, but it would be more effective if you would read through the exercise a number of times and then practice it a number of times so that you can do it anywhere, even without the audio equipment which would be necessary if you depend on playing the recording every time you want to do it.

To achieve its results, you first sit comfortably in a chair or on the floor or ground – anywhere that is comfortable, where you can sit for about twenty minutes or more.

Sit with your back upright, chin tucked in a little, eyes closed. If in a chair, put feet flat on the floor. If cross legged, sit in a comfortable way. If you cannot sit comfortably on the floor, but want to learn to sit cross legged, use a chair until you are able to do that without strain, and then on the floor once that is comfortable. You want to be able to sit without discomfort for the entire time of your meditation. In meditation you also want to stay alert so, for most people, lying down is not a good option because that usually promotes sleep. You are trying to achieve a relaxed attention.

Of course, if you have medical problems, you will have to adapt. I spent over four months immobilized on a hospital Stryker frame. In that condition, lying down was the only thing I could do.

If you are in a group, you may want to have one person speak the instructions for everyone else to follow, so that everyone is at the same stage in the group meditation. Group meditation is very powerful, by the way, so gather a number of people of like mind together, and try it. That will also create a community of friends who can share their common interests and concerns.

As you read over the following instructions, imagine you are doing what they suggest by visualizing as you read. That way you will quickly learn the pattern of relaxation here.

With eyes closed, adjust your posture and your breathing until you feel comfortable.

Move your attention to your face. Relax your face muscles. Feel the muscles around your eyes relax, then the muscles around your mouth, cheeks, forehead and chin. Once that is relaxed, move your attention to the top of your head. Relax the top of your head. Move the relaxation to the back of your head then to the sides of your head. Feel the relaxation around your ears then allow the relaxation to radiate to the centre of your head.

Feel the relaxation in your whole head.

Now move the relaxation into your neck. If there are any tense areas, consciously relax those.

Move the relaxed attention into your shoulders. Feel them relax.

Move the relaxed attention into your upper arms, then into your lower arms and into your hands and fingers and thumbs. Feel the relaxation in your arms again. If there are any tense muscles, tighten them and then release them. That will usually help relax them. Some muscles will require many sessions or even years to relax.

Move the relaxed attention into your shoulders again, and then gradually move it down into your chest and upper back: into your stomach and middle back: into your lower back and lower abdomen. Relax the buttocks and genital area. Then be aware of the whole of your body's trunk, relaxed.

Move the relaxation into your upper legs; into your lower legs; down to the ankles; into your feet and toes.

Now imagine that your awareness is flowing like warm water from the top of the head, down through the neck, arms, body, legs and feet into the earth below you.

Feel your whole body relaxed and grounded to the earth. Sense your oneness with the earth. At this stage your body may even feel heavy, as if it is being drawn by a force greater than gravity. Just enjoy the feeling of being one with the earth.

It is important not to "space out" while doing this exercise. Although it involves relaxation, it is not just a relaxation exercise. It is actually a way of making yourself aware of your body and everything in your body. This is the basis of the kinds of awareness we will work with later in this book. Jesus said that "The Kingdom of God is within you." This awareness exercise is where we start the process of discovering the Kingdom of God.

This progressive relaxation/awareness is the prelude to most exercises in this book so, when I say in later exercises, "Relax your whole body," that means to go through this series of relaxations. With practice, you will find it easy to relax, even in two minutes.

Now that you have a sense of relaxed attention in your whole body, you will find it easier to do the review of the day (or night) which you have been doing, because you will learn not just to relax, but also to focus the attention and the memory.

Using this relaxed attention, you will be able to see how the different memories of the day or night affect your body. You may find certain parts of the body become tense as you remember some things or you may be able to feel the emotions more vividly once you have gone through this relaxation process. This will help you to note the underlying effects of what has happened to you during the day or night, and this is what you want to become aware of.

Emotions or stress register strongly in the body, but we often find ways of repressing their effects. Once you have made yourself aware of the body through this relaxation process, they will be more obvious to you. Ideas or attitudes will also be reflected in your bodily awareness. As you combine the "awareness of the day" exercise and the "relaxed attention" exercise, you will find that your body is a mirror for the activities and feelings you have been involved in. You can learn a great deal about the deeper aspects of your being by observing the body.

The relaxation/awareness exercise and the review of the day and night may seem like merely a way of relaxing, but you will quickly find that you are uncovering what is really happening to you, deep within the areas you usually ignore. Because you are uncovering the hidden things in your life, you may be tempted to judge what you find there. Do not judge. You need to learn to be very gentle with yourself.

We are all sensitive to judgement and condemnation when it comes from others. We are even more sensitive to the judgement which comes from ourselves. It is important, then, as you sit in the Silence and as you become aware of any negative things which happened during the day or the night, to be willing to forgive yourself and others. The act of forgiveness allows you to perform the next stage of the daily meditation, after you have become aware of the things of the day – letting the day and its contents flow away so that you are free from them and can move forward without carrying a burden of guilt or anger or desire for revenge.

Nothing else is required at this point in your meditation. Just review the day and let what you find, flow from you, so that you are renewed every morning and night. If you become aware of something you specially like, just note it. If there is something you find negative in your experience, note that as well. Otherwise, let the things go. Do not hold onto anything.

You may find it valuable to write about your experience. Keep a separate notebook for this. Bring the events and insights of the day into focus, write them into the notebook, then enter again into the review of the day, then write and then enter again into the meditation. This "journaling" is often a way of creating even more clarity in the way you understand your life. It is also good to be able to look back over your journal from time to time to see what patterns and changes you see there.

Do not make resolutions to change too early in your practice. This exercise is for awareness. Change will often result from this awareness, but allow the change to grow from within instead of trying to force it through decisions of the mind. Allow your awareness of any event or emotion or idea to mature so that you see its effects over several days or weeks or even months – do not judge as soon as you see something you think is negative. Allow your awareness of your life to deepen over time and then allow the heart to make the decisions. Although the decisions of the heart usually take a bit longer to accomplish than the instant judgements of the mind, the decisions of the heart are lasting. Think of all the New Years' resolutions you have broken and you know how untrustworthy that kind of change is. Let the change arise from deep within.

When you have finished your review, say a brief prayer of thanks no matter what you remembered, negative or positive. You do not want to hide anything in your review and gratitude is very important in this process, as is honesty. Then let the concerns go from you and enter with gratitude into sleep.

Let go of guilt or shame or judgement or attachment or worry of any sort. Let go of plans and hopes as well. Remember that you will have another day to deal with those. Then sleep with the sense of God's Presence around you.

In the morning, on waking, sit or lie with eyes closed. Ask for God's Presence. Go through the progressive relaxation. Remember the night which has passed. Bring into memory whatever happened during the night, including any dreams. Then look ahead to the day. Don't try to plan in detail what you will do, but be aware of the general shape of the day. Bring any concerns or worries or hopes to God in prayer. Offer the day to God, trusting that the best outcome will arise. Then enter into the state of relaxed attention, allow your attention to move over different parts of your body and enjoy this time of relaxation and renewal before the day begins.

(Of course, if you work night shift, reverse the order of these exercises.)

As you do these exercises, try not to force anything. Do not strain to remember, do not worry if you cannot remember what you did and do not judge anything you see. Be gentle with yourself. ***The aim is a gentle awareness of how you are living your life.***

Becoming aware of judgement is very important. You will notice that, as soon as you judge, you shift yourself out of the quiet, detached awareness which came from the relaxation exercise. You may even find you have to do a quick progressive relaxation again to enter into the relaxed awareness. Gradually you will be able to move beyond the emotions, fears, prejudices, condemnation or judgement to a "higher" state of awareness. As you do this, you will find a new type of understanding growing in your life in surprising ways.

It is difficult to describe what this state will be like for you, but you will feel relaxed, you will begin to develop a sense of God's Presence around and in you, and you will begin to have a greater sense of peace in your life. This will carry over into the events of the day as well.

Doing this exercise regularly will gradually bring your life into a state of conscious living from a higher, spiritual perspective. There will be little "Ah-ha" moments, when you realize certain patterns of action, belief or relationship which have been causing problems in the past. You may suddenly become aware of some skill or ability which you had not really paid attention to before. You may even begin to discover that you "spontaneously" want to change some of your ways of doing things. This is the time for change -- not as a result of negative judgements about yourself, but as part of a growing realization of how you would really like to be – a realization of what your whole life looks like, not just what the little fragments look like.

***

Meditation Exercise: Identifying barriers and correcting errors

As you review the events of the day and as you become aware of the body, it is inevitable that you will find negative things in your life. Traditional Christian teachings call these negative things, "sins." In that context, sins are seen as disobedience against God and the punishment for sin, it is said, is death and damnation.

In the Prayer of Silence there are no sins. Anything which is negative, which causes disharmony, conflict or suffering, is called "error." There is no disobedience against God, either, because there are no laws to break. How can that be, you may wonder?

The Prayer of Silence uses Jesus' story of "The Prodigal Son" as the model for how we deal with errors. It is worth quoting that story here:

> Then He said, "A certain man had two sons. And the younger of them said to his father, 'Father, give me the portion of goods that falls to me. So he divided to them his livelihood.
>
> And not many days after, the younger son gathered all together, journeyed to a far country, and there wasted his possessions with prodigal living. But when he had spent all, there arose a severe famine in that land, and he began to be in want. Then he went and joined himself to a citizen of that country, and he sent him into his fields to feed swine. And he would gladly have filled his stomach with the pods that the swine ate, and no one gave him anything.

But when he came to himself, he said, 'How many of my father's hired servants have bread enough and to spare, and I perish with hunger. I will arise and go to my father, and will say to him, 'Father, I have sinned against Heaven and before you, and I am no longer worthy to be called your son. Make me like one of your hired servants.'

And he arose and came to his father. But when he was still a great way off, his father saw him and had compassion, and ran and fell on his neck and kissed him.

And the son said to him, 'Father, I have sinned against Heaven and in your sight, and am no longer worthy to be called your son.'

But the father said to his servants, 'Bring out the best robe and put it on him, and put a ring on his hand and sandals on his feet. And bring the fatted calf here and kill it, and let us eat and be merry: for this my son was dead and is alive again: he was lost and is found.'

And they began to be merry. (Luke 15:11-24)

In the Prayer of Silence this is taken as the model for the relationship between us and God. The father in the story represents God and we are the son. The son goes into a far country and wastes all he has in riotous living. When he comes to himself, he thinks he has sinned, and he tells his father he has sinned, but his father will not even listen to that kind of talk. The father does not think the son has sinned against him or that he deserves punishment. Rather, in love, the father welcomes him home, knowing that, in his heart, the son has already changed.

That same pattern is what is followed in the Prayer of Silence, knowing that God has already forgiven us – in fact, God has never condemned us, so we do not have to fear.

The Prayer of Silence is built on a completely different idea of what we call "evil," than that found in the major monotheistic religions of the world.

In order to account for evil, they have asserted the existence of a second god, one almost as powerful as the first, who is the source of evil, to be defeated only at the end of time and the world. Time and the world are thus seen as the "realm of Satan." The defeat of Satan necessarily becomes the end of the world and of time in this way of thinking.

But in a truly monotheistic religion, there is no Satan who is the opposite of God. What we know of as "evil" is not something opposed to God, but rather an expression of the freedom which is also an aspect of God. All souls can choose the destructive path – the path of anger, hatred, violence, jealousy, murder and the like. In this they do not oppose the "Will of God," but choose that path for a time until they learn its results. When they finally understand where this "left hand path" is leading them, most souls will choose to follow the path of love.

Souls choose their own suffering until they learn the path which delivers them from suffering. Neither path is "evil," – it is just that some actions lead to suffering and some lead to union with God.

In traditional religious thinking, the mind is split and helpless until Satan is defeated. In the Prayer of Silence, the mind is split until it becomes aware, in itself, that it is better to follow the way of love rather than the way of hatred. Deliverance and "Heaven" can be found in time and in the world because "the Kingdom of God is within you." We do not have to wait till the end of time to start setting things right in our lives and our world.

What others call "sins" we call "error" or "ignorance." Error can always be corrected and ignorance can always be remedied by learning truth. There is nothing here which deserves punishment, and punishment has no part in the Prayer of Silence thinking.

When you do find something in yourself – some fear or anger or hatred or other negative thing which is causing a lot of problems for you or for others with whom you are related– there is an exercise you can do which will get rid of most of the problems you have to deal with. This exercise will give you the pattern for working with what Carl Jung called the shadow side of your nature.

Many people think that Sigmund Freud was the person who discovered the unconscious, but there is a passage from one of the alternate gospels which suggests that Jesus knew a great deal about the unconscious almost nineteen hundred years before Freud.

In *the Gospel of Thomas* in the *Nag Hammadi Library* (discovered in 1945 in Egypt), Jesus is quoted as saying to his disciples:

"If you bring forth what is inside you, what you bring forth will save you. If you do not bring forth what is inside you, what you do not bring forth will destroy you."

Here is one of the best descriptions I have seen of the effects of not dealing with negative subconscious feelings. You really do need to "bring forth" and deal with the negative things within you, or else they will destroy you. Note also that Jesus does not say that God will punish us for what we leave undetected within us. It is the negative thing itself which will destroy us.

When you have identified a negative aspect of your life which really needs change, you will have to spend some concentrated time working on resolving the difficulty. In order to devote the necessary time to this process, find a quiet place to sit where you will have time to explore the negative feelings or actions or thoughts you want to correct. Close your eyes and do the progressive relaxation you already know about. Let the tensions fade from your body. Ask for God's help. Then do one of the following exercises to achieve a detached perspective.

***

Just talk to God about it:

The first way which may work for you is to talk with God about each item you want to correct. You can even imagine you are the Prodigal Son come back to the father and you want to discuss with him what has been going wrong in your life. Talking to God will help you to move beyond self-condemnation, to an attempt to understand and find healing. Make it seem as if both you and God are looking at the problem and discussing it. With practice you will find that you will get an answer from God. It will come in words which form in your mind.

With your eyes closed, let your mind move over the issue you are faced with. Let's pretend it is a fear of some sort you have to deal with. You can imagine God asking the questions and you giving the answers. What are you afraid of? Do you know when the fear began? How does it make you feel, specifically? Do you feel like running and hiding? Is it a focused fear or is it more general? Do you feel like attacking whatever you are afraid of? Ask whatever questions seem appropriate.

Continue the questions until you have a well rounded sense of the source and effect of the problem you are dealing with. You want to achieve a sense of distance between the problem and who you are. You are not the problem. The problem is an error, not a sin, and so is not something which is actually a part of your nature. The problem is something which is added onto you, and you want to get rid of it.

Once you have the error in focus, it is time to commit to correcting whatever is wrong. Tell God you no longer want to hold onto the error. Ask God to correct the error and wash away any effects of the error.

***

Treat it like a person:

Another way to distance yourself from the problem is to treat it as if it is a person, separate from you. Once you have entered the Silence as usual, you will be able to sense the problem manifesting somewhere in your body, in pain or discomfort or tension.

When you have found the source of the problem, talk to it. You can say something like, "I know you are afraid. Why are your afraid?" When it answers in your mind, continue the conversation. Allow the problem to speak fully. Do not argue with it or contradict it. It wants to be heard, so let it talk to you. Even encourage it if it is afraid or angry.

Most inner problems will act as if they are a person if you speak to them. I call them "proto-personalities," because, if they are left to develop, they can become part of your personality. You can become a frightened person or an angry person or a greedy person if the proto-personality becomes dominant. On the other hand, if you deal with the error, you can become a more loving, honest person.

After you have talked to the difficulty for a while and are quite sure you have it in focus in your mind, you must make a commitment to get rid of it. It is not sufficient to think that maybe you want to get rid of it. Be sure. Also, do not start to feel pity for the proto-personality. It is not a real person. It is merely the way a particular problem has taken on the qualities of a person.

Once you have decided definitely that you want to be rid of the problem, ask God to help you resolve the error and learn from it. Use simple words which are honest. Do not feel you have to use complex prayers. Remember how Jesus referred to God as "Abba" which is the Aramaic word for "Dad," and talk to God as if you are talking to a very familiar, down to earth, loving Divine Parent.

Once you have asked God for correction, concentrate on your breathing and, as you breathe, let the difficulty flow out of you with the out breath and feel a sense of new, cleansing life entering with the in breath.

I initially found I needed to breathe twelve times, in and out, in order to let go of things I had held onto for a long time. Gradually, I found that I could reduce that to seven breaths and then to three and then two breaths. But even now, if what I am correcting is a major error in belief or feeling or attitude, I will sometimes go back to the seven breaths to let it go completely. Experiment with this.

***

Remember, there are three steps in this process of correcting any difficulty:

1. Enter into the Silence in the usual way and then become aware of as many aspects of the difficulty as possible by bringing it into focus in the mind. Use one of the methods above to get a sense of distance between you, as a person, and the difficulty, which is merely an error in your approach to life.

2. When you feel you have the problem in focus and are ready to let it go, you can ask God in prayer that it be removed from you. If you like, you can "will" or "intend" it to go. This can be done with a variety of words. Find a phrase which seems to suit you, like "I am ready to let this go. I correct it/ I ask for divine help in correcting it/ please correct it, God."

3. Finally, let it go as you breathe it away. In this act you turn it over to the divine creative power which is within and around you. Visualize it flowing from your body and dissipating in the air around you as you breathe. It was a destructive influence in your life and now you want to allow it to dissolve.

If there is still some error left after doing this exercise, repeat the above process. Very often our problems have multiple layers, like an onion, and we cannot let them go all at once.

It is important to become aware of this method of correcting error in yourself, since we will be using it frequently in the future. Again, do not think of your actions or attitudes as "sins" which must be "atoned" for. Think of the father in the story of the Prodigal Son, and be willing to bring your errors to God, knowing that you will be accepted and that the errors will be corrected. God, like the loving father (or mother), is even waiting on the road for you to return to a more wholesome life.

This process may take several sittings, and some of the difficulties may hang around in different forms for many years, but at least you will have them in the open AND you will have begun a relationship with God based on honesty. You will not start by hiding your doubts or the negative things in you, to have them come up over and over from their lurking places.

You are not in this for instant results. It has taken a long time to get where you are now, and it will take a while to get where you are comfortable with God and with your inner self, but at least you are going in the direction of honest discovery.

It is also important, at the end of your meditation, to say thank you for what you have experienced or perceived. Gratitude puts a seal on what has happened and welcomes the new state of being as a vital part of you.

You will have become aware by now that part of the Prayer of Silence is directed at finding peace within, but finding that peace also involves discovering things about yourself which need changing to make it possible to continue in that peace. The same goes with love. You want to find love within but, in order to do that, you must overcome all those things which get in the way of love.

In a sense, this is a kind of psychoanalysis without all the analysis. Your main focus is on developing the positive things within you through daily meditation. The "analysis" part comes in whenever you find a problem in your inner nature which needs to be resolved. It need not take a lot of time to resolve the negative. You want to spend most of your time on a relaxed awareness of your day and night and how God is part of that daily life. You want to develop and build the positive you find within yourself.

You will also discover, if you open and close each exercise with a simple prayer, that this practise will gradually make you aware of the Divine Presence within the events of your life. It will be a subtle realization, so don't look for anything dramatic. Some people may have dramatic experiences, and that is fine. But do not become attached to dramatic events. Let them go with gratitude and continue to seek the growing, subtle change of awareness which comes from deep within you as you grow in everyday spiritual perception.

***

The simple practises suggested in this chapter will also make you aware of three of the central ideas in the Prayer of Silence, about consciousness and how it creates the world around us.

1. *All that we are and all that we have around us arises from within.* We are like magnets, attracting to us more of what is within us. Until we begin to become conscious of our lives, our perceptions are often dense and opaque, so we cannot see what our experiences really mean as reflections of our desires, hopes and fears. We do not realize why we attract to ourselves the things we do. But the daily awareness exercises will gradually make us conscious of the causes of our lives.

2. *You will gradually begin to see how the Divine Presence can actually be a part of your everyday experience.* Most people think of God as being like one of the opaque and dense events of their lives. As you include God in the daily review of your life, you may find that you spontaneously begin to talk to God during the day in a completely informal way. This is the conversation you can expect to arise at some time, gently, informally, in a friendly way. Gradually, without pressure or striving, you will become aware of the intimate relation to God of which Jesus spoke when he described God as "Abba, Father" or which Elijah experienced as the "still, small voice" of God. Allow this to develop. Do not try to force this to happen, but be aware that it is a natural part of your growing life within the inner Kingdom of God.

3. *The Prayer of Silence is similar to what the early church called "Practising the Presence."* This is an "Awareness Meditation," because it involves a process of becoming aware of as much about ourselves, our ideas, emotions, relationships, beliefs, fears, hopes, abilities, potentials and loves as possible.

"Practising the Presence of God" is the centre of this form of meditation. We bring ourselves to the stage where we can actually feel the Presence of God within and around us: and we become aware of the way the rest of our life is an expression of that central core. A later chapter will be focused entirely on Practicing the Presence.

In the early stages of meditation, it is difficult to focus because of the distractions of everyday life. Most meditative traditions have a way of promoting focus in meditation. In the early stages of the Prayer of Silence, focus is achieved by giving the mind something specific to focus on. First you focus on the events of the day. Then you focus on the body and on relaxation. Then you focus on any of the changes which you want to make in your life. All of this achieves the same thing which focusing on a "mantra" or on a flame or a sound does, but it also helps build a balanced life at the same time.

As you continue to meditate, you will begin to discover an inner peace which is its own focus. If you are focusing on the events of the day and then become aware of this peace surrounding you, let go of the events and focus on the peace. The same is true if you feel the joy or love which sometimes well up from deep within you. Let go of the more mundane affairs of the events of the day and allow yourself to be absorbed in the joy or love. Later, I will suggest other ways of promoting focus to continue to move you toward more advanced spiritual states of being.

In advanced meditation, it is possible to enter the peace of the Presence of God quickly, in almost any setting. You can let the world slip from you for a time, trusting that the things of the world will be waiting for you when you return, but that you do not have to concern yourself with them in the time you have devoted to the Silence. In advanced meditation you will be able to switch quickly between the "two worlds" of the Silence and your everyday life. You will learn to find fulfilment in both.

Both the beginning and the advanced student of this Prayer are aiming at the same thing -- the awareness of the Presence of God within and around them. When you are advanced, you will be able to sit silently with God and share whatever you wish to share with God and know there are no barriers keeping you apart. Getting there is largely a matter of learning what to do with the errors you experience within yourself and how to become immersed in the love, joy and peace which arise from your spiritual centre. But even the beginning student can find peace in the Presence of God, even if only for a short time each day.

It takes quite a bit of work for most people to get to the advanced stage on a consistent basis. We have built up many barriers over the years. In the Silence we are gradually cleansed of fear and anger, hatred and jealousy, greed and lust, judgment and condemnation, violence and theft, attack and defence and all the other divisive, destructive things in our lives. In their place, like roses sprouting out of manure and rotting compost, grow the beautiful flowers of truth and honesty, generosity and loyalty, forgiveness and fellowship, sharing and encouragement, compassion and love.

Your progress in the Prayer of Silence is measured partly by how much of the negative you are able to leave behind and how much of the positive you are able to cultivate. However, there is a paradox here, and the paradox centres on judgement, that thing we are involved in on many levels. Unfortunately, we tend to condemn ourselves when we discover the negative things which the Prayer of Silence quickly uncovers. Judgement cripples us because, in condemning ourselves, we make it difficult to go beyond condemnation.

You want to be able to leave behind the negative without judging, but it seems like you have to judge in order to know what to leave behind. You need to develop "awareness without judgement," knowing that when you are fully aware of the effect the negative has on your life, you will automatically leave it behind without judging yourself or others. In the same way, when you become aware of the positive things in your life, you will want to develop more of those, again without judging yourself or others.

***

I want to make a shift just here. As you will find when I tell you a few stories in a later chapter, I have come to know Jesus as Yeshua. The name "Jesus" is derived from a Greek form of his name. "Yeshua" was his original name.

The name, "Jesus," has acquired many associations and meanings over the years in many churches and religions. The name "Jesus" is related to many doctrines and beliefs which we will find ourselves leaving behind in this practice of the Prayer of Silence. For this reason, and to leave behind all of those associations at the very beginning, I will call Jesus "Yeshua" in the rest of this book. You will begin to develop different associations with that name, associations which do not carry all the baggage of the other traditions. Also, many people have picked up negative feelings and attitudes associated with the name "Jesus" as they were growing up.

I remember one person from a conservative background who was told when he was a child that every time he did something wrong, he "put another nail in Jesus' hands." It was very difficult for him to deal with the negative things he found in himself because of this early training. Changing the name back to the original "Yeshua" will help people like him overcome this kind of association.

This will also make you aware of the importance of early childhood experiences as you confront some of the negative things in your review of the day and the night. Most of the time, you will want to just be aware of any things you discover, without judgement. However, when you find they are troublesome, or when you are aware of a pattern in which they are showing themselves to be "proto-personalities," which are affecting your life, then you can go through the cleansing exercise you have just learned – again, without judgement.

In the same way as you can develop a relationship with God as "Abba," as Yeshua did, so too you can develop a relationship with Yeshua. He is alive, and is able to help you in many ways when you ask. So, as you continue the daily time in the Silence, allow yourself to develop a sense of Yeshua's presence with you as well.

It is important to stress something about "worship" at this point. This may seem like a surprising thing to say, but it is important not to worship God or Yeshua. The act of worship always puts God at a distance from you. I have learned through much experience that God does not want to be at that kind of distance. God is not "high and lifted up;" somehow far away from us. God is to be found in the inner sanctuary of our own inner being. There we can "talk to God as a man talks to his friend," as Moses did. And Yeshua is not to be worshipped either. He is our "elder brother" in spirit, and we need to cultivate that sense of a close relationship, not the distance which worship brings.

Again, it may take some time to overcome the kinds of training we have had about the act of worship, but it can be done. If it is a big problem, talk to God about it, as in the above exercise, and then let it go and enter into a closer relationship with God than worship makes possible. The intimate relationship which you can develop with both God and Yeshua is something you will come to value more than anything. So work toward that. Even in a "worship service" you can let others treat God and Yeshua as if they are far away, but you can enter into the Silence and feel their presence with you in your inner being.

**

In order to know God, the Prayer of Silence teaches that we must first begin to know ourselves. Yeshua teaches us to pray, "Our Father who art in Heaven," but he also teaches, "The Kingdom of Heaven is within you." It is, then, as we come to know what is within us, in the Heaven of our Spirit, that we begin to discern the Presence of God.

As we become "knowers of God," we also begin to discover things about ourselves and our lives which can lead to a greater fullness of life within us, our communities and our world. From that God-focus, many other benefits and responsibilities flow. In the prophetic tradition of the Bible, there is always a very strong emphasis on mercy and justice. The act of meditative prayer is first of all for our own spiritual growth. But the prophetic tradition teaches that we cannot stop with our own development. Inner prayer should make us sensitive to the needs of others so that we can gradually develop a spiritual society, concerned with the needs of others. That does not mean that we will take over political power, but that our inner attitudes will be reflected in the societies we produce.

Once we see God in ourselves, we will also see God in others and we will want for others what we have for ourselves. Yeshua emphasized many times that "in as much as you help one of the least of these my brothers and sisters, you help me." In the beginning stages, it is often difficult to be concerned with the needs of others, because we think that helping others is taking something away from us. We will find in advanced stages that all people are extensions of our being so, in helping others, we are actually helping ourselves.

***

The Prayer of Silence and religious traditions:

It is almost impossible at the beginning of the twenty-first century not to have heard of some style of meditation. Although some people and organizations have condemned meditation as a "New Age Phenomenon," with the implication that it is merely an upstart fad, the roots of meditation go deep into our past as a human race.

We need only look at the sources of some of the many forms of meditation, to realize that almost the whole world is represented in those roots. You may have heard of the meditative traditions of Sufism, Zen, TM, Yoga, Kundalini. The Sufis are a mystical group within Islam, originally from the Middle East; Zen originated in Japanese Buddhism; TM, Yoga and Kundalini have their roots in India, in Hinduism. When the Dalai Lama fled Tibet in 1959, he also brought a now quite popular form of Buddhism with him. Buddhist meditation is now quite commonly known over much of the world, with Buddhist temples in most large cities and some Buddhist meditation techniques used even in many churches.

Increasingly popular healing arts like Chi Gong and T'ai Chi (from the Chinese Taoist tradition), Reiki (which originated in Japanese Buddhism), Therapeutic Touch (from a North America research scientist), the Laying on of Hands (from the Christian tradition) and many others, are becoming known as ways of meditation, exercise and healing. The number of meditative and healing systems has exploded in recent years, with healing by people like Drs. Kam Yuen, Richard Bartlett and others seeming almost miraculous.

With the opening up of the world to inter-continental travel from the 18th to 21st centuries, the publication of sacred texts from many countries and the great movements of people around the globe, there has been a sharing of ideas and experiences, so that people of all faiths and cultures have profoundly in-fluenced each other.

Ironically, the Christian meditative tradition is not so well known as the oriental variety in the contemporary church, where meditation has often been looked upon with some suspicion as an "artificial" or "forced" way to God. The argument in some churches is that we can not possibly do anything good enough to warrant salvation. Therefore, salvation has to be purely an act of God. We should try to be good people, but ultimately our salvation depends on what appears very much, in some theologies, to be God's whim -- called God's Grace, by some -- which is unpredictable and might fall on anyone and omit anyone; or Adoption, where God decides to adopt one person but not another; or Election, where the Elect are chosen before birth and the others are damned from before birth.

I have known several people who were raised in these traditions, who had lived very good lives, helping others and living morally, but were terrified when death was coming close because they said they could not know if they had been "chosen" by this apparently arbitrary God. They could not trust in God's love, they thought, because their churches taught that the doctrines were stronger even than love. In that context, meditation really finds no place at all, because everything depends on God, and they believe that nothing the person does can have any effect on the outcome.

Some churches have adopted a few, isolated meditation practices from a variety of meditative traditions – a little silence here, a little chanting there, the ringing of a bell during prayer once in a while and a little concentrating on the breath at some other time. But as far as I know, there is no consistent use of meditation in Christian churches, because it is difficult for most Christians to see how meditation fits into their world view. There is even an undercurrent in many Christian churches which argues that effort in spiritual disciplines is wasted, because our fate all depends on an unpredictable God. Therefore, instead of seeking to perfect our inner person in relation to God, they say, we should be making sure we believe the right list of doctrines so we can get into Heaven.

The Roman Catholic orders, the Quakers and the Eastern Orthodox churches have had meditation as part of their practice for many years, and there are some rich resources in those areas, but even there (with the exception perhaps of the Quakers) correct belief and correct doctrine has been much more important for salvation than any attempt to open the gates to the inner Kingdom of God through meditation. Meditation by the laity has even been forbidden many times in history.

In most Christian churches, believers are taught to practise correct belief (and less often, correct action) in order to get into Heaven or Paradise, a distinct place where souls go to live only after they die. In that context, meditation can be seen only as a minor variation on the idea of "prayer," not as a complete life guide for spiritual growth. Usually, in Christianity, beliefs and doctrines are the core around which all other practices are clustered, and "spiritual growth" is only a minor feature of the Christian life, where correct belief, with its related development of intellectual study, is of most importance.

As far as I know, this book, and the system of spiritual growth which it outlines, is the only complete and consistent guide to spiritual growth in the Christian tradition, the only book which presents in detail a complete and consistent theory and practice of spiritual development. And it has been able to present such a coherent account of the role of meditation in spiritual development because it is based on a complete rethinking of the meaning of the Christian message.

Drawing on biblical roots, the teachings of Jesus, personal experience, scientific observation and practical examples, *The Prayer of Silence* presents a comprehensive theoretical basis for the description it gives of the development of spiritual awareness.

It offers exercises, appropriate to each stage of growth, for developing the key aspects of spiritual consciousness, and it presents ways for enhancing positive awareness and for dealing with the negative aspects of experience, encompassing all aspects of spiritual, intellectual, emotional and social life.

It takes a radically different approach to the ideas of the relationship between God and humanity, and to the nature of spiritual consciousness and the intent of the teachings of Jesus. Again, as far as I am aware, it is the only book which presents a complete, practical system for achieving the Divine Union which Jesus envisaged when he said, "I and My Father are one. . . I am in My Father, and you in Me, and I in you. . . but you know Him [the Holy Spirit] for He dwells with you and will be in you" (John 10:30; 14:20&17).

The Prayer of Silence sees "Heaven" as a condition of consciousness within us, not a place we go when we die. It is therefore important to develop this spiritual inner "Kingdom of Heaven" in order to draw closer to God while we are in the body, so that we can continue our growth in the same Heaven after the body dies. We carry Heaven with us as part of our inner nature.

The Prayer of Silence derives much of its power from the realization that there is no death, because the Spirit is always alive, even after the body dies. And the Prayer of Silence also stresses that we are never lost, never put into an eternal place of torment, because spiritual suffering is merely an aspect of our inner nature which can be healed as we seek God's Presence within us. The fear associated with Hell and eternal punishment is the product of a religious materialism which takes changeable, inner states of being and says they are eternal physical places.

Rather, the Prayer of Silence teaches that we are given the freedom to explore all conditions, even those where we have chosen to live very negative lives. When the time is ripe, we, like the Prodigal Son, will "come to ourselves," we will realize the effects which our acts have had on others and, having experienced those effects in our own lives, will repent and decide to return "to our Father's house" to live in love.

We are never trapped in any "eternal" state of suffering, since there are no eternal states. The Spirit in constantly in motion, "like the wind," Yeshua said. As we enter repeatedly into the Silence of God, we become aware of how the Spirit moves and where it moves. The Holy Spirit and our Spirit are not just confined to the Earth and Heaven. They can move into many conditions and can do many things in all realms, as you will discover. Through all of this change, our Spirit will finally learn the major lesson that it can be one with God, as Yeshua was one with God.

God is not far away, either. Like the father in the parable of the Prodigal Son, the Divine Father, Abba, is always waiting on the road for us to return. The son does not have to hold right beliefs about the father: the son merely has to decide to return home, to take the journey back to his father's home. The way to this Kingdom is to seek transformation within ourselves. As we turn from the negative things which keep us from the Divine, we begin to experience God's Presence within ourselves.

In Yeshua's teachings, God is not unpredictable, either. Yeshua tells us that "all who take the sword will perish by the sword," (Mat 26:52) and "You will know them by their fruits. Do men gather grapes from thorn bushes or figs from thistles?" (Mat 7:16). St. Paul says something similar: "Do not be deceived. God is not mocked: for whatever a man sows, that he will also reap" (Gal 6:7). Yeshua even goes further to tell us not to judge others at all, "For with what judgment you judge, you will be judged; and with the measure you use, it will be measured back to you" (Matt 7:2).

There is Law in our moral lives and our relationships, and we must live by it. The foundation of the law of cause and effect is love, since the aim of this law is that we eventually learn love and union with God. We have freedom to try out any life we want. There is one proviso, however: We cannot bring great suffering to others and then repent and think we have escaped. To fully learn the lessons of our actions, we must experience in our own souls what we have brought into the lives of others. Once we have done that, then we can fully appreciate the implications of our actions.

Finally, we will learn from our successes and our errors, and eventually we will learn wisdom and understanding and compassion. It may take a long time to get there, but that is the aim. This law of cause and effect is similar to the now well known Law of Karma. This law, that we must reap what we sow, is the basis of all the preaching of Yeshua and the prophets -- Amos, Isaiah, Jeremiah, Elijah, Ezekiel, John the Baptist -- they all told people that if their living was wrong and if they did not change, they would have to face the consequences, because the effect always arises from the causes in human behaviour.

The negation of human responsibility and effort in seeking "salvation" or spiritual understanding, in a number of churches, is not consistent with my reading of the Scriptures. My experience in many years of seeking God's Presence is that God would like us to be much more active in perfecting our relationship with others and with God. Yeshua uses very active words to describe our search. We should "knock" and "seek" and the door will be opened and we will eventually find what we are looking for (Mat 7:7).

Yeshua even tells us, "Therefore you shall be perfect, just as your Father in Heaven is perfect" (Mat 5:48). I am sure he would not have said that if he thought God was going to pick and choose who was saved and who was damned, and if he thought that effort was not worthwhile. We are supposed to be like the woman who turned everything in her house upside down looking for the lost coin (Luke 15:9), rather than the unfaithful servant who buried his coin because he was afraid of his master (Mat 25:25). Responsibility for our actions is essential in Yeshua's teaching.

Yeshua even compares the Kingdom of God to the widow who kept pestering the judge until he gave her what she wanted (Luke 18:6). That widow is what we should be like, because we have to show God that we are serious in our search for spiritual awareness -- we must keep trying, even if we do not get what we want the first time. Yeshua seems to be saying, "Work at this: it does not come easily and it does not happen the first time you try it. You have to keep following the path in order to find your way home."

There is a very important principle here. Our lives are lived by habit and it is very difficult to change habit. Just think how hard it is to go on a diet and then STAY on a diet or how difficult it is to give up smoking or any other bad habit.

What we are doing here is even more difficult than a diet, because we are changing things which are fundamental to our way of living in the world. Many people will try meditation for a few days or weeks and, when they do not get the instant results they are used to in matters of ego gratification, they will give up and say, "See, I told you it wouldn't work." Or they may say that entering the Silence of God does not help them to understand and accept doctrines, so they are not interested. They may even say that they really need an intermediary between them and God, so they will go back to the priest or other person who can tell them what to believe and how to behave. For them, the Prayer of Silence is laying just a little too much responsibility on their shoulders.

We really do need determination to make the Prayer of Silence work. It is interesting that many Eastern teachers of meditation will not accept Western students because they say Westerners expect instant results and the teachers know that, in spiritual matters, nothing is instant. It really does take hard work and perseverance to succeed in spiritual pursuits and this is true for a very good reason.

Again in parable form, Yeshua says something very important about the spiritual life, "And no one puts new wine into old wineskins; or else the new wine will burst the wineskins and be spoiled, and the wineskins will be ruined" (Luke 5:37). Wine used to be put in skins, not in bottles. New wine continued to ferment for a while, causing expansion of the new wineskins. Once the wine became mature, it would stop expanding and the skins would harden. There was no elasticity in the old skins so, if you put new wine in the old skins, they would explode and the wine would be lost.

Meditation is difficult for your own protection. Your emotions, beliefs, ideas -- and even your body -- change and grow as you meditate. If you are "hardened in your ways" and try to change too quickly, you will find that the new perceptions will almost literally "burst your old skin of beliefs and ideas." People complain that spiritual growth is slow, but that is for your own good. If you do not take time for this change to occur, you will cause damage to your whole system because the change will happen too quickly and your body and emotions and ideas will not have time to adapt. You must not rush what you are doing.

Some people have argued that psychedelic drugs should be used for spiritual growth because they are so much faster at opening the inner awareness. However, most people who have taken that road find that, although the the drugs do open the inner doors, they open them too quickly, so that all the negative things come pouring out as well, all at once. These "bad trips" can be very destructive because they make the "wineskins" burst. And even the "good trips" are arrived at so easily that the other qualities of strength, balance, perseverance and insight, which usually come with gradual growth and reflection, do not come when drugs are used to try to develop spiritual vision. This is because meditation does not just bring visions. It also changes the whole person to accommodate the new, underlying understanding of the spiritual life.

Allow the new awareness to grow gradually without judgement or hurry. There is no rush. Enjoy the new perceptions and allow yourself to become accustomed to each small change before pushing on to the next. It is better to integrate change into your everyday life over a long period of time, to make sure that the change will be beneficial and permanent.

***

Meditation Exercise: Awareness of the moment

This meditation exercise is related to the twice daily exercises you have been doing. It will develop further the awareness which is growing in you as you do that meditation.

Note that in all these exercises you are not just relaxing. They are to make you aware. In fact, these exercises are all helping you to develop a type of awareness which most people do not experience.

You will also realize by now how this book is organized. Since you need to develop both the theoretical and the practical aspects of the Prayer of Silence at the same time, I provide alternate passages of theory, followed by exercises, then more passages of explanation, then more exercises. What you think and believe affects deeply the experience you will have, so I provide alternate ways of thinking about the spiritual life so that you can begin to see your experience in a new light.

***

This exercise will help you to become aware of your daily life from a different perspective, one that will enrich many aspects of your experience once you become conscious that it is possible.

Like the morning and evening review exercises, the time required for this exercise is not great. You will only need a few minutes a few times during the day.

In this exercise, you will be expanding your awareness in new ways, because instead of just reviewing your life twice during the day (continue to do that while doing this) you will begin to extend your awareness to the immediate "now" of your experience. You will have both the comprehensive awareness provided by the morning and evening review, as well as an awareness of how your life unfolds through individual actions, decisions, words, conversations, thoughts, scenes and experiences.

It is important not to turn this exercise into a continual analysis of everything you do during the day. That can be destructive, in that an analysis will involve evaluating, judging and trying to determine how your life should go and will take you away from actually living your life. *Do not become obsessed with observing yourself.*

In this exercise you are actually not observing yourself at all. You are observing the world around you. The aim of this exercise is again a gentle awareness, with the emphasis on "gentle." Do not judge. Do not analyse. Do not try to put things into words. Do not try to force change.

And do not do this all day long. This is an intermittent exercise, a couple of times a day, when you stop the flow of events and consciously become aware of what is around you.

I will give examples to illustrate how to do this.

***

In a natural setting: Usually, when we go for a walk, our minds are filled with many things – the worries of the day, what a particular person said, how we could have done something differently, what we have to do in the evening. Our focus is on ourselves as we follow the constant inner chatter of the mind. This exercise will allow you to move out of that chatter for a few moments.

In this exercise, then, you are going for a walk. Stop somewhere and look around you. Do a quick progressive relaxation, starting at the top of your head and moving down to the bottoms of your feet. Allow your mind to move through your body, relaxing every part of your body in a matter of seconds without closing your eyes or sitting comfortably. Now, briefly allow your awareness to focus outside yourself, on things around you – things like the leaves on the trees, the sounds of the birds, the feeling of the wind on your face, the rustling of the grass and the colours of the flowers.

When you first start doing this exercise, you will be using your physical senses but, with practice, you can gradually develop other senses. Try to get the feeling that your awareness is not only coming from your senses, but that it is moving out horizontally from your back and your body, pushing farther and farther out until it envelops the world around you. Feel everything around you being incorporated into your being, so that you begin to feel, for a moment, that you are one with the world you perceive. It is as if you have a spiritual body which has expanded and is now surrounding everything around you. It is perceiving by surrounding everything in its perceptual field.

Just be aware – nothing else. Do not put anything into words. Do not name things. Try to move beyond word-shaped perception to a non-verbal awareness. Keep this awareness for as long as is convenient and for as long as you can without the inner chatter of the mind taking over. Do not strain to do this. Be relaxed and merely enter into the life which is taking place around you.

When the words and ideas start up again, return to the body without regret and say a word of thanks to everything around you for whatever perceptions you had. Do not try to analyse what this is about. Just enjoy the perception. You will begin to understand its purpose later, but the understanding will not involve a lot of words, so I will not put a lot of words here to describe it.

***

In a crowd: You can do this exercise where there are people as well. Being aware of a crowd with this exercise is very interesting. Everything seems to slow down – but I will not say what happens. Just try it.

When we are in a setting with other people, we are usually concerned with how we appear to others, whether we are liked, whether our hair or clothes look just right, whether we will be able to speak without others criticizing us and other ego concerns. In this exercise you focus outwards, away from yourself, as in the nature exercise above. You move away from ego concerns to perceive the world without the ego involvement.

With eyes open, move your awareness through your body, relaxing it very quickly. Then move your awareness outside of yourself to perceive the world around you. You will discover when you do this, you are not really observing what is around you with the senses. It is more like you project your awareness outward to surround everyone in your awareness.

You will sense what people are saying, how they are saying it, how they are interacting, how they seem to be feeling toward each other, how they position themselves in relation to each other. You will sense the furniture or the walls. Your awareness is moving beyond your personal, ego concerns to an awareness of the dynamics of human interaction. The aim is not to judge others but just to be aware of them.

As you do these exercises, you will gradually feel yourself expanding into the things around you. This is almost literally a spiritual expansion because it is not just your senses perceiving things in this state of awareness. You are actually expanding your spiritual presence in the landscape or the room.

In the morning and evening meditation you are making yourself aware of your body and then of the events of the day. Your consciousness there is focused on you and on how you interact with the world through time.

In this exercise, you are doing something different with your consciousness. You are making yourself aware of something which some scientist have discovered about perception. Our perceptions and our senses operate in a field of awareness. Our bodies occupy space but our senses seem to be able to move around in that space in a way bodies cannot. As you do these exercises more and more you will find that the space occupied by your awareness will grow larger and, with practise, you will find that you become aware of things around you which are not even discernable to your physical senses. You will begin to make contact with other "spiritual fields" in this way. You will develop some very subtle spiritual senses.

Again, don't judge or analyze. Just be aware.

Continue to practice the morning and evening meditation because it is developing some important aspects of your awareness. Then, two or three times a day, introduce this new exercise which will gradually help you develop a multi-level awareness, one in which the life of the world, with which you are familiar, becomes enriched with a growing awareness of the spiritual dimension of living, with the Kingdom of God which is within and around you.

Chapter Three

Place, Time and Values for Deeper Meditation

"But you, when you pray, enter into your closet, and when

you have shut the door, pray to your Father which is in secret,

and your Father which sees in secret will reward you openly"

(Matt 6:6)

This is a very short chapter but deals with some essential housekeeping items about the life of prayer and meditation.

In the New Testament there is very little information recorded about Yeshua's approach to prayer. The disciples even complained about this so, we are told, he taught them what has become known as "The Lord's Prayer," "Our Father which art in Heaven." However, even though it is recorded that he did not teach them much about prayer, Yeshua actually told his disciples some very practical aspects of prayer. Given the nature of what is recorded, one wonders if he taught them about meditation, instead of the synagogue prayer which was common among the Jews of his time. Perhaps he did not teach them what they expected, so they thought he was not teaching them about prayer.

For instance, he told them where they should pray – and the place he told them to set aside for prayer is really only suitable for some form of meditation. He did not tell them to pray in the synagogue or the Temple in Jerusalem. He told them, "But you, when you pray, enter into your closet, and when you have shut the door, pray to your Father which is in secret, and your Father which sees in secret will reward you openly" (Matt 6:6, RSV).

You are supposed to pray in your closet!

You have likely already discovered that you do need a place set aside for prayer and meditation. We are told that Yeshua often went to the wilderness to pray, to be away from the crowds. And if you want to go much further in meditation, it will be necessary for you to establish a special place, as well as a particular time, for your regular meditation.

When you really look at what Yeshua was saying, you will find that he was telling his disciples, "Find a small space, an inner space, where you can meet with God in private on a regular basis. If you really want to enter into a close relationship with God, the kind I have, you need to be able to meet with God in secret. And God, who sees what is in secret, will answer you."

Part of the reason you need to make a conscious choice of a place for meditation is that it indicates to your deeper self and to God that you are serious about what you are doing. You are not just doing your spiritual work when it is convenient for you to do so. You are committed to an intentional practice. You have decided to devote time and place to what you are doing. It is important. It is a part of your life to which you are devoted.

Soon, I will be leading you into some forms of meditation which will take you deep within yourself and you will need to have a place and time where you can be quiet and alone to devote those twenty minutes twice a day to communion with God in your inner being. If you want to go further in this, you really do need to make such a commitment.

The place you choose should be as private as possible in the beginning, although with experience you can enter the Silence anywhere – I have meditated very deeply on a rattling bus in India, driving over a very bumpy village road with so many people, and chickens, sitting and standing in the aisles that it was impossible to move, let alone fall over. However, to develop the skills to be able to do that, you need to start with a definite place and time, if at all possible.

But there are some good psychological and physical reasons to have a regular place to meditate. If you use the same place over and over, it becomes familiar enough so that you can forget about the place, the outer environment, and you can concentrate on what is happening within you. You do not have to continually adapt to a new location. Your chosen place becomes the "Prayer of Silence place" and, when you enter that place, you know it is consecrated for one purpose, at least during the time you are in the Silence.

Some people like to have a few sacred objects or pictures to remind them of their purpose. A picture of your "guru" or teacher is sometimes helpful. Perhaps a picture of Yeshua would add to the atmosphere. Maybe some objects which have special spiritual meaning for you, will add to the atmosphere. In that case, you are creating a small chapel, which is not a bad idea at all. Try not to make this place too cluttered, though. Keep it simple. The aim is to draw the attention into your inner being, not out into the environment, even if it is a sacred environment.

Having a desk and table available was, and still is, important for me, since I often record in my journal any important perceptions which arise in my meditation. The simplicity is also important for me, but I know that some people like a bit more ceremony than I do, so having sacred items in your meditation space might actually help you to concentrate on your task.

In the 19th century, when a lot of Spiritualists were developing their mediumistic abilities, people discovered that having a "cabinet" helped them concentrate their energy. Often, the cabinet was exactly that – a piece of furniture that was specially made just large enough for the person to sit in comfortably with adequate ventilation, like a closet. They discovered that they tended to build up peaceful "vibrations" in that place. If you meditate in the same place every day, you will achieve the same effect. The place itself begins to become peaceful so that the more you meditate in one place, the easier it becomes.

The closet, as Yeshua suggests, might be just the place you need, if you can arrange it appropriately!

One woman told me that she booked up the bathroom for her time of Silence because, with four children and a husband, that was the only place available in their busy house! Of course, everyone else had to arrange their other functions accordingly. When you think of it, a storage closet or a study or a little used basement room or shed or corner of the back yard or a barn or a bench in the local park or a hill or forest or cave might be just what you need. Some people use one corner of the bedroom, set aside as the "holy spot."

There are many possible places, depending on your lifestyle.

Do you have a favourite chair to sit in, or do you know how to sit yoga fashion on the floor? If you are not well, lying on a bed or sitting in a wheelchair might be a good alternative. I mentioned before that many years ago I spent almost six months in a hospital bed with a broken back, and since then, lying on my back has been a very good way to meditate. I have learned not to fall asleep.

***

Relationships:

Unless you are living alone, you will have to come to terms with the changes which meditation makes to your relationships. You are asking others to accept that you are going to be taking about twenty minutes twice a day out of your schedule, but that will impact on the time commitments of others in your household.

It is important to try not to take over time which has been very important in your relationships: waking or going to sleep with your spouse, for instance, or activities with your family members. Be sensitive and negotiate times which would be mutually acceptable. I made it a practice to get up early, meditate, and then return to bed so that I could wake with my wife, since that was an important time of sharing and of starting the day together. Even then, there were adjustments which had to be made. I found that 3:00 a.m. was actually a good time to meditate. It is a very peaceful time, when the whole world seems to be asleep, and it is traditionally a fruitful time for spiritual insight.

You can agree with other family members that you are not to be disturbed while meditating. I phoned a house once and a small voice said, "Mommy can't come to the phone right now because she is meditating. Can you call back later?" Turn on the answering machine if you have one. Your twenty minutes of Silence is more important than taking every phone call.

Many years ago I visited a home where one of the family members used to sit in meditation in the middle of the living room. No one else was allowed to use the room while she was there and everyone had to tiptoe around the house or she would get angry at them. This was very counter-productive. If she had withdrawn to a bedroom and closed the door, the problem would have been solved but, in this case, it seemed like she was more interested in making a statement about her meditation than in finding inner fulfilment.

Perhaps others would like to join you in meditation, but do not be pushy in this. The Prayer of Silence will bring changes in your life and will have an impact on others -- with sensitivity they can be positive for all concerned, but do not insist that everyone in the family do the same thing you are doing. If they see that it has been good for you, perhaps later they will join you. If you make it a source of conflict, they will not be interested at all.

***

Meditation Exercise for establishing time and place

As with most major decisions, it is helpful if you meditate on what you have to do before finalizing your plans. That way you create an inner image of what you want to achieve and you imprint your plans on your total life vision. Any major decision can be examined and affirmed in this same way. You will quickly begin to realize this is a very effective way of introducing new things into your life.

To imprint time, place and relationships in your mind, enter the Silence in the usual way, going through a progressive relaxation, surrounding yourself with the light of God and asking for God's guidance.

Visualize yourself in the place of your choice at the time of your choice. Sense this time and place in as much detail as possible, even if you are not in the chosen place while you are doing this exercise. Consider any relationship issues which might arise, one person at a time, including the people who might seem the most insignificant. You may uncover some issues in this way which you had not seen while in your usual state of consciousness.

Once you have all of this in focus and you are sure you want to go ahead with your commitment, ask God to help you establish that time and place as important parts of your life. You will be imprinting them on your idea of how your day should function. When you are finished, surround yourself with light and God's Presence and say a word of thanks for what you have received.

You may find you have to work into the new schedule gently and sensitively. For instance, if you have chosen the place your children love to play in, then it would be good to change place instead of fighting with them. If it becomes a cause of conflict and anger, you have defeated the purpose of the new time. Be gentle with yourself and be willing to experiment with other times or places which might be better. Always ask God for help in overcoming any conflicts.

If you find later that the time or place or the relationship issues are not working out as you had hoped, re-examine the whole thing and find an alternate solution. Enter meditation again to establish the new time and place as part of your life pattern.

Imagination is very effective in the spiritual life, and the active form of imagination, visualization, will become extremely important in the exercises we do later in this book. Everything we do starts in some way with imagination. Then we manifest what we have imagined. Even huge bridges or sky scrapers or ships start with imagination. By exploring all of this in a meditative state, you will actually be changing your inner time and place orientation so that you will create the conditions which will make it possible for you to practise your meditation regularly.

Remember that your lower ego, which has a lot of investment in power and position and your present habits, will try to create difficulties for you and others. You may also find you have to overcome a kind of spiritual pride which wants to exhibit your "spiritual superiority" to others by making your spiritual practice public and obvious.

Some people will even find themselves creating conflict with others in order to show both their holiness and their martyr complex. Many people who are interested in spiritual things have this martyr complex, in which they actually want people to persecute them. They WANT people to give them a difficult time about their spiritual practice. They want others to persecute them so that they can demonstrate how superior they are.

As strange as it may seem, in the early centuries of Christianity, the church in several cities in the Roman Empire actually had to prohibit Christians from actively pestering the authorities so that they would be thrown to the lions. This martyr complex is a very common part of the spiritual personality. If you find yourself doing anything which provokes others to persecute you, meditate on the problem and correct it as in the earlier exercise designed to correct errors.

Remember Yeshua's words with which we began this section. You do this in secret, so that your Father, who knows what is in secret, will reward you. This meditation work is not designed to make you look good to others. It is designed to develop your inner, secret relationship with God. Work with sensitivity and commitment and honesty and be willing to adapt and change as you perceive more about yourself.

Be aware that the inner room and the time of meditation are only partly about actual physical place. Mostly they are about a state of mind, about a commitment, about a sense of withdrawing into the privacy of the self, about establishing a place to meet regularly with the divine within you and about finding your oneness with God, apart from the chatter of the world of the ego.

***

Values

Yeshua also taught some fundamental values which were necessary aspects of the spiritual life. He knew that the Prayer of Silence did not come about by accident. It is an intentional act. You decide to do it and, as with all things you decide, you need to evaluate if you have the resources to carry it out.

So Yeshua said to his followers,

"For which of you, intending to build a tower, does not sit down first and count the cost, whether he has enough to finish it – lest, after he has laid the foundation, and is not able to finish, all who see it begin to mock him." (Luke 14:28-29)

To achieve the Kingdom of God we must develop certain ways of perceiving, but we also have to develop certain qualities in ourselves. Yeshua knew very well that it is always easy to start something but that it takes a particular quality of life to finish it. The Kingdom of God requires perseverance, understanding, commitment and honesty.

Yeshua also knew that the spiritual life was not easy and, in planning for our life of the spirit, we have to recognize that it will require a lot of our interior resources to complete. After all, he compared planning for the spiritual life to building a tower, a difficult and expensive structure to build. You are not building a chicken coop.

Related to the parable of the tower is another parable – the parable of the sower. In this parable Yeshua spoke of other qualities we need if we want to develop our spiritual lives. In this parable a farmer is sowing seed in a field in the ancient way, scattering it by hand from a bag:

"Listen! Behold, a sower went out to sow. And it happened, as he sowed, that some seed fell by the wayside; and the birds of the air came and devoured it. Some fell on stony ground, where it did not have much earth; and immediately it sprang up because it had no depth of earth. But when the sun was up it was scorched, and because it had no root it withered away. And some seed fell among thorns; and the thorns grew up and choked it, and it yielded no crop. But other seed fell

on good ground and yielded a crop that sprang up, increased
and produced: some thirty fold, some sixty, and some a hun-
dred." And he said to them, "He who has ears to hear, let him
hear!" (Mark 4:3-9)

Notice that in this parable Yeshua even tells his audience, "Pay attention! If you have ears, you had better listen!" There is obviously an important lesson here.

In this parable are the different qualities of those who hear the teachings about the Kingdom of God and react in different ways. Some of these are warnings of possible weakness. Others are qualities Yeshua would like his followers to develop.

Some people hear the message but do not pay any attention to it -- so it does not even sprout in them. It is like seed which has fallen on rocks.

Some people are like shallow ground where the soil is warm and the seed germinates and grows quickly. These people are initially very enthusiastic and are the sorts of people who want to be actively involved in the spiritual work right away. They want to convert everyone else as soon as they have been converted themselves. However, when the heat of the day comes and difficulties arise, they wither and die because they have no root in what they are doing. They have not bothered to develop a deep understanding of the message of the Kingdom of God.

Some people have the message choked by different types of thorns and weeds. They give in to family or social pressures, they "do not have time," they "will get to that later in life" and so they cannot grow because of their concern about what others think. They have no root in themselves.

I initially wrote, "But there are always the *few* who hear the word and bear a good crop according to their ability." Then I realized that, when a farmer plants his field, he expects most of the seed to sprout and bear a crop. Yeshua was actually optimistic in this story about how many people would respond. He must have felt that many people would respond to his teaching, so that the field would be filled with a good crop. In later teachings, he talks about the bountiful harvest which will be ready when the time comes, and then he will need labourers who are willing to go into the harvest to reap the rich crop.

But it still requires inner strength, a fertile field and deep roots, to be able to commit to one thing for a long enough time to find results. Those who will really grow in spirit have a deeper root than most, a greater sense of persistence, a realization that something really must change in your life and that this Prayer of Silence is providing you with an opportunity to find that change and to learn of your spiritual nature. Even if you do not initially have this quality, you can develop it if you really desire to do so.

Perseverance has its rewards. If you have gotten this far, and if you have done the exercises in meditation, your life has changed. Even just reading the book will change the way you see things.

You are now living life more consciously, on many levels. You have discovered some important things about yourself. Setting aside time every morning and evening has helped to give focus to your life. The relaxation exercises will help your body and your emotions to heal. Correcting any errors you find will make your life more balanced. Practicing the exercise where you project your awareness into your perceptual field will make you aware of things you did not know about yourself before.

All of this will make your life richer and more productive. All of this is good. I am aware, however, that, for many people, this may be all you want. And that is okay. You have made a start on the inner path. That can never be taken away from you. You have learned something new which will change you forever. You can continue to live consciously in the light God gives you in your time in the Silence and you will continue to grow.

You may already have produced a crop of thirty percent, as the parable says. Not everyone is ready for sixty or one hundred percent. Become conscious of your abilities and work with them. Do not judge or condemn yourself just because you have not gotten as far as someone else.

It is possible, however, to go much farther in our inner quest if we want to and if we feel we have the resources to do so. And it is here that we need to evaluate several things about ourselves and our practise in order to decide how much time and effort we wish to devote to this inner growth. We have to decide whether we have the resources to build the tower. We have to decide whether we will bear a crop of thirty or sixty or one hundred percent.

There is no condemnation if you decide not to build the tower or if you want to bear a crop of thirty percent. Just be honest with yourself and do not measure yourself against others. You are the one who is involved here, not others.

There is a helpful tradition which comes from the Hindu religion. In that religion there are ideally four stages in life, and even then, not everyone achieves all four. People are expected to start out as students, devoting their time to learning. Then they become "householders," people who devote their time to raising a family. Following that, the ideal life expects the person to become a "man (or woman) of affairs," someone who will give back to the community through service to others. When they have completed that phase of life, they renounce the world and become recluses, people who devote all their time to the spiritual life.

Of course, not everyone can do all of these things, but there is a sense of proportion in this ideal, in the realization that different people in different phases of their lives seek different things. Not everyone is on the same part of the path of life at the same time.

That is why it is important not to compare yourself with others but to evaluate where YOU are in life now, and how much time and effort you can devote to this spiritual practice at the present time. If you have family or other responsibilities, it may not be possible for you to devote a lot of your time to the Prayer of Silence just yet. But even a little bit of effort in this regard can enrich your life, and when the time is more appropriate to pick up your practice again, you will have already achieved a lot of insight into life and relationships.

***

Meditation Exercise: Evaluating where you are on the spiritual path

In order to evaluate where you are in terms of the commitments you want to make to the spiritual life, it would be helpful for you to enter the Silence as usual, ask for God's guidance and then bring into your mind all the questions about what you should do with your spiritual life at this point. Be honest, knowing that there is no condemnation in whatever choice you make.

Ask God for help in determining what your priorities should be. Then sit in the Silence and wait for things to clarify themselves. Share any concerns which arise until you have come to a conclusion about your level of commitment. When you are satisfied with your results, thank God for what you have received.

My case is likely an extreme case. I had the Death Experience in 1966. Then in about 1979 I began a concentrated program of meditation in order to heal a number of ailments which were causing me a lot of trouble. After I had been meditating regularly in this concentrated way for over a year, around 1981, Yeshua came to me in my time in the Silence and asked me if I wanted to enter a "training project." He said it would be difficult and would require all of my inner strength, but that it would be worth it in the end. He said I could stop anytime I wanted if it got too hard.

I thought about the offer for quite a while. Did I have the inner resources? Would I be able to "finish the course," as St. Paul puts it? I finally said I wanted to be part of this training. And it was difficult – the most difficult thing I have done in my life. But it has been the most valuable thing I have ever done, as well.

Writing this book is bringing me close to the end of the most difficult part of the training project. But it was from going through this training that I have been able to learn a great deal about my inner nature. I was able to heal a broken back and severe brain damage caused by encephalitis. The result has been that I have been able to write this book which can make it a little easier for you and others. I have gone over the path first to find the difficult spots and to learn the means of overcoming those difficulties.

As you go farther into the Silence, you will also find that you are asked to confront what you are within – the negative and the positive. If you have tried to change any negative things in your life, you will already know that it is not always easy.

But the Prayer of Silence offers ways of dealing with the negative aspects of your inner being, transforming them into positive growth. It allows you to take the hurt and betrayal of the past and turn it into love. It is a powerful means of transformation. It also helps you to identify the positive abilities which can be activated through inner work and it makes your life fuller and more balanced.

In evaluating whether you want to go further on the spiritual path, then, remember that there are many resources here in this book, and there are those in spirit who will also help you. You are not expected to do all of this alone. My path may have been hard, but I had Yeshua and Abba with me all the way to help me achieve the level of spiritual understanding I have.

Not everyone has a lot of trauma in their past, but if you are a person who has some very dark things in your life, you will benefit greatly from practicing the Prayer of Silence. Just a brief description of some of the people I have helped will give you an idea of the kinds of darkness which can be faced successfully with the Prayer of Silence.

There was the man who grew up in Nigeria during the civil war. He had seen such horrors that he only felt safe in a building with walls four feet thick and a steel door. He was able to overcome his fear and live a more trusting life.

There was a woman who was raped and went through an abortion and was condemned and disowned by her Roman Catholic family. She was able to overcome her guilt and separation from her family and was able to be reunited with her mother who had disowned her.

A young man who was close to suicide because of the expectations and condemnations of his father was able to learn to live according to his own values and develop a life measured by his own sense of success.

A member of one of my meditation groups was an eighty year old woman who felt she had never had a childhood because, from the age of eleven, she had to look after her arthritic mother and all her younger siblings. She was able to enter in meditation into the reasons for her experience and find resolution to the conflicts and sadness which made her later years so difficult.

Not everyone has these kinds of experiences to deal with, but these are the kinds of things many people have to face in life, things that they carry around with them all the time. Even if the areas of darkness in your life are not as serious as these, it still takes inner strength to deal with them and it is for this reason it is necessary at some point in a program of spiritual growth that we stop to evaluate whether we have the resources to deal with all we are. The good news is that the Prayer of Silence, with its gentle, gradual approach, surrounded by the Love and Light of God, can provide the necessary support to get through even the most horrible experiences.

You see, this Prayer of Silence is not just about bringing you nice, fuzzy feelings. It is about giving you strength in a world which requires strength. The world is not easy, as you know. In fact, the world can be terribly hard and painful and lonely. It does, however, become meaningful when you are able to see it in the light of the "other world," the inner Kingdom of God, to which you have begun to gain access through the simple meditation exercises you have learned so far. The Prayer of Silence can give you a whole new world of meaning in the midst of the difficulties of life.

Be honest with your feelings when you talk to God. You cannot get anywhere by trying to sugar-coat your real reactions to what you have perceived in life. If you would succeed in finding your way into that secret place where you can talk to God as to a friend, you must be honest.

I know from my own experience of tremendous suffering that there is light at the heart of even the deepest darkness. But it often takes tremendous faith to be able to face the darkness and allow it to be healed by the Light. In what follows, I will give you specific instruction how to deal with the darkness, but it would be irresponsible of me to tell you that everything will be happiness and light all the time, when I know, from the experience of many people, that you will have to deal with the shadow side of yourself in meditation.

However, most people are aware there is darkness within them, and they are looking for something which can deal with it. People have told me how the "feel good" philosophies have failed them and how the Prayer of Silence has finally made it possible for them to deal with their troubles and find meaning in their lives.

It is for this reason I include a lot of exercises for dealing with difficulties in the inner way.

***

Love, Joy and Peace:

Finally, in talking about the values and decisions which will make it possible to move further on the spiritual path, it is important to realize that this way is not all difficulties. As you confront the negative within you and seek healing, you will come to greater wholeness. In fact, you will discover that, hidden behind the curtain of darkness, is a Joy and Love and Peace which "pass understanding." You will begin to discover the bliss which comes from finding the Divine nature within you and within others. You will begin to act out of love and creativity in ways you could never have expected.

As you become experienced in the practice, you will find that the exercises and suggestions mean more and more each time you do them and that the positive experiences in meditation will spill over into your everyday life in wonderful ways. You will also discover your own creative ways of dealing with challenges along the path because, once you embark on a serious quest, you will discover that you activate spiritual help from within and around you. You are not alone in this. God is active in the relationship. There are beings (which have been called "angels" or "guides" in many traditions) who are assigned to help us in our search, if we will only call on them for assistance.

So, in planning the building of your spiritual tower, do not just evaluate your own resources, but take into account the divine spiritual resources you will find in the inner way. That is where faith in the testimony of those who have already gone over the path helps tremendously. You will find meaning as they have.

***

Let me tell you about some of these people who I have seen change and then you will have a better idea of how this might affect you.

I have a colleague at the university where I teach who was an atheist. At one point in his life he came to the conclusion that life had no real meaning, until he started to meditate; meditation introduced him to a world he never suspected was there, in spite of all his training, and now he tells me how this new awareness has completely changed his approach to his research, teaching and life and has made him much more compassionate as well as much better as a researcher and teacher.

I know a woman who was an alcoholic and had lost her husband and her children and her job before she started on this way of Silence. Since entering that profound confrontation with herself, she has finished two university degrees and is making a great contribution as a counsellor of troubled children.

Another person, who had cancer and was a member of a meditation group I led in our church, feels that meditation helped bring her through the trauma of cancer and contributed to her remission.

I know a man who had Lou Gehrig's Disease (ALS) and, as the disease progressed, found in the assurance of the practice of meditation the strength to find meaning even when dealing with that very difficult disease. It was a profound privilege to be able to talk with him and have a small part in helping him through his difficulties. He derived tremendous strength from his inner awareness and lived many years beyond the time the doctors had given him.

And there are so many more – all of them seemingly ordinary people who found extraordinary strength and beauty in their lives because of the Prayer of Silence. They would all say that meditation has changed them radically, but they also feel that is what they needed and continue to need.

Remember, if you do decide to continue to sit in the Silence of God, you will be joining the company of an increasing number of people around the world. We seek to move beyond our own limited resources as we grow toward a greater sense of God's real presence with us.

Chapter Four

A Dweller in Two Worlds

"My Kingdom is not of this world." (John 18:36)

Yeshua knew he was from somewhere else, even though he was also from this world. "I want you to be in this world but not of this world," he said. These kinds of comments, about living in two worlds, have always been a mystery to me. What exactly did he mean by that kind of statement? It was as if he lived in two worlds and saw both of them clearly. What is it to be a Dweller in Two Worlds? In 1966 I had a Near Death Experience (which I will describe below) in which I actually entered into a different world. Was that what Yeshua was talking about, I wondered?

I want to introduce you in this chapter to some strange things: To Yeshua's often obscure teachings about what he called the Kingdom of God; to what the ancient Greeks called *"Gnosis"*; to an idea from India about an aspect of our being called "Atman"; and to a level of our own consciousness which I discovered when I died in 1966, and which I call the "Watcher."

These ideas are all related to each other and will prepare you for your own initiation into your own Watcher level of consciousness, and into the powerful uses to which that can be put.

One of the most important things I learned during my Near Death Experience (NDE) in 1966 was that death is not really a physical event at all, even though it has physical consequences. Later I learned how death and meditation are very similar. For the person who dies, death is merely a shift in consciousness, in the same way as meditation is a shift in consciousness which you have been practicing every morning and night. Both meditation and death give us admission into another realm of being. But that has another implication. That means that birth was also merely a shift of consciousness, from a state where we did not have a body to a world where we do have a body.

The next level of the Prayer of Silence is quite different from most types of meditation because it is designed to make you aware of your eternal nature very quickly – more quickly than most methods. It makes you realize that you really are a Dweller in Two Worlds.

Before I introduce you to the Watcher, I must explain a number of ideas, and tell you some stories which will prepare your mind for what happens when you actually go through your "initiation" into this new awareness (in the next chapter).

Once I have provided this background and have introduced you to the experience of your Watcher consciousness, you will be able to practice almost right away, what it has taken the great spiritual masters many years to accomplish. That is not to say that this will be easy, but it will help you to enter the land of Spirit much more quickly than usual. That way you will be able to go farther into the Silence of God than would be possible otherwise.

It is necessary for you to learn this speeded up version because human spiritual evolution must itself be speeded up for our own survival. We are at a point in our history where we must change radically or we will perish. The global problems we face are extremely serious and appropriate economic, political, environmental and religious changes are impossible unless people learn how to change themselves from within. It is necessary to get as many people as possible to learn of the benefits of entering regularly into the spiritual states learned in the Prayer of Silence (and in other methods of meditation now being taught around the world), so that we can transform our earth.

This prayer, then, is not practiced just for selfish reasons. Personal change must be seen as a prelude to change of society and the world.

Much of what I teach here is based on Yeshua's parables. However, I will introduce you to a different understanding of his ideas than that normally taught in the churches. Yeshua taught his disciples "secret knowledge." He had to keep much of this knowledge hidden in his time because it was forbidden to reveal too much of it. It is now time to let many more people into the secret.

***

God is like Yeast!

Yeshua taught some strange things. People over the years have tried to make them acceptable to as many people as possible, but they are still strange. They can be read as simple moral teachings. Powerful institutions have transformed them into doctrines and beliefs and have even taught fear and fought wars to bully as many people as possible into believing their interpretations.

However, it is possible to look at his teachings differently. They can actually be seen as clues to a great mystery in the human spirit, and that is how we will approach them in what follows here. You may not have been introduced to this strange, mysterious side of Yeshua so, just for a little while, sit back and enjoy a trip through a different world. I will explore a number of ideas in the rest of this chapter. It may not be obvious right away how each piece fits into the puzzle but, by the time we get to the end, you will understand.

Our first clue to the meaning of the mystery Yeshua taught his disciples comes when he says, "My Kingdom is not of this world" (John 18:36). That has been said so often that it has lost its bite. But he meant it literally.

"There is this world that you see around you all the time," he might have said. "It is a world of power and possessions and violence. You want me to be a king in this world, like King David, but I refuse to be your king. My kingdom is not here. It is somewhere else entirely."

He tried to take his disciples into this different world through his teachings but, over and over, they could not understand what in the world he was talking about. Like the good, moral folk they were, they tried to make his teachings apply only to the world they were already familiar with. They turned his teachings into moral messages and doctrines, because that is what they already knew. What is familiar always seems the safest. His followers found it terribly hard to move beyond what they were used to into what he was trying to teach them.

Over the years of exploring the spiritual realms in the works of many of the great Masters of Spirit in many traditions, I have discovered that Yeshua knew a great deal about the spiritual realms – what he calls his "kingdom." I call this aspect of his teachings "spiritual psychology." Churches and religious groups do not seem to be aware that much of his teaching had to do with the nature of this "spiritual psychology," this inner world, instead of the doctrines, beliefs or moral laws which they teach. As we saw earlier in the passage from *The Gospel of Thomas* about the necessity to bring hidden things to the surface so we can change them, Yeshua knew a lot about the subconscious.

I started my life wanting to be a minister in the United Church of Canada, but gradually found that what I really needed was "a religion that works," not all the theology and doctrines which seemed so empty of real meaning. It would appear from the number of people who claim to be looking for "spiritual" rather than "religious" meaning, that many others are in the same situation I was. I wanted a religious truth which told me something about my inner being. I wanted a spiritual practice which would help me actually live my life, not just tell me about someone else's theories about life.

I searched for many years, but it was hard work. None of this comes easily, as you who have searched know. The inner being is mysterious, and finding your way through the inner streets, alleys and paths is far from simple. Initially, it is even difficult to get an idea of what an "inner kingdom" might look like.

As I was led farther into my inner self through a number of experiences I will describe below, and as I became aware of a whole inner kingdom of the spirit, I realized that many of the obviously weird teachings recorded as coming from Yeshua, were actually clues to the nature of our inner being and were not meant to be turned into doctrines or moral laws. They described, in a hidden way, the aims and experiences of the inner spiritual search. They had more to do with the Quest for the Holy Grail than with the Ten Commandments.

The problem with Yeshua's teachings is that he didn't want most people to understand him and the meaning was actually meant to be hidden. Most preachers and theologians speak as if Yeshua really wanted people to be able to understand him. But what Yeshua himself has to say on the subject emphasizes that the relationship between people and God will continue to be a great mystery for most people, in spite of his explanations. He did not want it to be easy to understand what he said. What he taught had been hidden for a long time and he knew that only a limited number of people would be able to understand.

The disciples had their teacher right there with them, but even they were obviously puzzled by what Yeshua was trying to tell them. From this distance in time, it is no wonder we are puzzled, too. In reply to his disciples' question of why he always taught in parables that few seemed to understand, it is reported that Yeshua even said, "Because it is given to you to understand the mysteries of the Kingdom of God, but to them it is not given" (Matt. 13:10). He says here that he teaches in parables in order to keep the mysteries mysterious. It is clear from the texts that the disciples didn't understand, either.

When we actually listen to Yeshua, it is obvious we are dealing with more than beliefs and doctrines which are designed to get us into a Heaven in the sky when we die. He wants his disciples to struggle with his teachings, to try to figure out the "mysteries of the Kingdom of God" which are hidden in his words. And to make it more complicated, the Heaven which Yeshua talks about is not in the sky at all, nor is it after death that we enter it. Churches and leaders of other religions have been able to frighten their members into obedience by threatening them with Hell if they did not believe their doctrines, and Heaven if they were obedient, but that was not Yeshua's concern at all.

What Yeshua called "The Kingdom of Heaven" or "The Kingdom of God" is a state of awareness into which we can enter right here and now. And Yeshua is not the first one who taught it. He refers often to the tradition of the prophets who went before him. Like Yeshua, the prophets also kept these teachings secret so that they would not be distorted by the masses of people.

You see, the spiritual realms about which he tells stories, require work and devotion to enter. They require study and knowledge and commitment. In some traditions it is said that the gates to the various levels of the Heavens are even guarded by fierce dragons or lions and only the truly committed can pass. We know from the previous chapter how important commitment is. You do not learn anything on the spiritual path without it.

Unfortunately, many people, perhaps most people, weren't willing to put effort into learning the real truths of the inner kingdom so, in the "schools of the prophets," there were always requirements for initiation into their mysteries. One such school, the Essenes, even had complex initiation rituals and periods of probation before you could learn the hidden teachings. Yeshua got himself into difficulty because he taught their secrets openly. But even though he told the stories openly, understanding Yeshua's teachings and entering what he calls the Kingdom of God or the Kingdom of Heaven, is not easy. It is certainly not a simple matter of saying, "I believe. I'm saved."

But let's take a closer look at his teachings.

The spiritual psychology which Yeshua taught states that we live in two worlds. There is the outer world in which we usually live – the one where his followers wanted him to be a king. We seem to be surrounded by this physical world and are bound to it by our senses, emotions, ideas and beliefs. Most of us could not say, "My kingdom is not of this world," as Yeshua did. Actually, our kingdom IS of this world, and we discover that it is a thoroughly unreliable world at that.

We have a very uncertain identity within this physical world. We are defined by our economic and social status, by our race and sex, by the beliefs with which we were raised, by the health of our bodies, by the weather, by our families, our neighbours and enemies. But all these conditions can change in a flash. This world changes all the time and is a place where, as Yeshua says, "moth and rust destroy and where thieves break in and steal" (Matt. 6:19). In fact, when this is our only world, we find that life is often frightening, empty and meaningless, especially when things begin to get difficult, as they always do some time in our life.

But, Yeshua says, there is another world which runs parallel to this physical, uncertain one. It is this other world which is the Kingdom of God. It is difficult to describe until you have actually experienced it, and even then it seems to be something he can only hint at. Yeshua had some stories with which he tried to describe the indescribable. I also have stories that I will recount which I hope will bring this Kingdom of God into focus for you.

It is not much wonder that the disciples had such a difficult time with Yeshua's teachings. They were ordinary men and women -- fishermen, tax collectors, violent men, workers, housewives, business people, prostitutes and the general riff-raff of society. They were very much of this changeable world and it was hard for them to look into the other realms and understand what Yeshua was talking about or even accept that there might be something in his ideas which related to them.

As Yeshua taught this band of unlikely followers, it is as if he is saying to them, "Let go of your preconceived ideas of what the spiritual realms are like and listen to some stories. Maybe from them you will get a little sense of what I am talking about, because I can not define it in the way that the priests in the temple define the laws you are supposed to follow. In my Kingdom there aren't any laws or doctrines to follow."

I do the same thing in these pages. You do not have to do anything just now except read the stories. Gradually you will get a glimpse of what is behind the strangeness of these tales. But these are more than just stories.

The first disciples heard these stories and tried to fathom their meanings. For them, as for us, these stories are actually part of an initiation into the mysteries of the spiritual kingdom. The first disciples even felt that finding the meaning of the teachings would somehow admit them into a whole new world of the spirit.

In *The Gospel of Thomas*, from which we quoted before, the writer, Didymos Judas Thomas, says, "Whoever finds the interpretation of these sayings will not experience death," (Marvin Meyers, Translator, *The Gospel of Thomas*. HarperSanFrancisco, New York, 1992.) This Judas Thomas was known to the Syrian and Egyptian churches as the twin brother of Yeshua, the one who, after Mary Magdalene, knew most about the mysterious side of Yeshua's teachings. Judas Thomas says that salvation is to be found in understanding the meaning of Yeshua's stories, not in having the right beliefs. For him, salvation is sort of like solving a puzzle.

If you want to enter that other world, the Kingdom of God which the original students of Yeshua sought, you must do as they did. Read, listen closely and pay attention until the meaning gradually grows within you.

Later I will take you through exercises which will make it possible for you to actually experience what these stories are trying to describe. You will learn what it is to live both in this changing world as well as in the spiritual kingdom. You will gradually become a Dweller in two Worlds.

Central to this spiritual psychology is the claim Yeshua made, "The Kingdom of God is within you" (Luke 17:21). If you are looking for meaning, do not expect to find it in the world around you. Look inside. The meaning you seek is within you.

In this Prayer of Silence you have been learning ways of looking within, ways of entering the inner Silence. You will learn to move beyond what most of the spiritual texts call "darkness," into what they call "light." The terms "light and darkness" may seem vague now, but as you enter the Silence regularly, you will discover that there actually is an inner darkness and an inner light. Perhaps you have even experienced some of that already. They are not just convenient symbols of good and evil. They describe states of consciousness which are very real.

Yeshua told a variety of stories about what this strange Kingdom of God is like [I paraphrase in the following passages].

"The Kingdom of God is like a woman who lost a coin and then cleaned her whole house looking for it. When she found it she invited her friends and celebrated with them" (Luke 15:9).

"The Kingdom of God is like a man who discovered that there was a valuable pearl in a field. He sold everything he had and bought the field so he could have the pearl as well" (Matt. 13:46).

"This inner kingdom is like salt which gives flavour to food (Mark 9:50). It is like yeast that causes bread to rise (Matt. 13:33). It is like a rich man who went into a far country and left his wealth with his servants. When he returned, he judged his servants on how well they had invested his money" (Matt. 25:14-30).

The Kingdom of God is obviously something invisible yet vital, like salt in food or yeast in bread. It seems vague and undefined, but when we find this lost "something," it brings tremendous joy or love or peace or wisdom with it, and we want to invite all our friends to share it with us.

"Seek first the Kingdom of God," he said in another place, "and then all the things of the world will be added to you" (paraphrase of Luke 12:31). "But," he went on to say, "if you only seek the things of this world, that will be all you have, and into the bargain you will feel that great sense of emptiness and meaninglessness which the world can never fill. What is the value in gaining the whole world," he asked, "if you lose your own soul?"

That sounds good, but what does it mean to "seek the Kingdom of God?" How are we to even begin the process which will clarify what this is? As you will see, the Near Death Experience I had in 1966 began to give me some clues about what all of this vague talk might mean. After all, for four months I could do nothing but lie on a narrow frame bed and think. Movement within my physical world had been limited to being rolled over every two hours by two nurses. Any activity I wanted to be involved in was limited to activity of the mind. I was forced to explore the inner world as most people never can, because I was prevented by my medical condition from exploring the physical world.

For a long time after I came back from my Near Death Experience in 1966, I found these stories of the Kingdom of God fascinating but frustrating.   I somehow knew that the essence of Yeshua's teaching was to be found in these sayings, but they seemed so general it was hard to figure out what he was trying to teach his disciples. In fact, they seem so divorced from our everyday experience that I wondered if they had to do with life after death. Yeshua does say at one point, "Let not your heart be troubled: you believe in God, believe also in Me. In My Father's house are many mansions; if it were not so, I would have told you. I go to prepare a place for you. And if I go and prepare a place for you, I will come again and receive you to Myself, that where I am, there you may be also" (John 14:1-3). Yeshua is talking about dying here. Does that mean that the Kingdom of God can only be found after death, as some people preach?

Yeshua never comes right out and says what this Kingdom of God is. It is always so vague, this thing we are supposed to look for. As most of you know, you who have searched for meaning beyond this world, it can be very frustrating because it is so subtle, as if it is there, but just out of reach.

But the most frustrating thing is that we don't even know what we are looking for aside from some nice symbols – yeast, salt, coins, pearls. And

Yeshua tells us that children and harlots and sinners will enter into the Kingdom of God before the righteous people. That does not even seem fair! He had "prostitutes and sinners" as disciples and was in constant disagreement with the Pharisees who were very concerned with applying the Laws of God to everyday morality, family values and politics. The Pharisees actually sound like good church people, the ones who want to lead a good life according to the Scriptures. So why would Yeshua object to them?

Whatever this Kingdom of God is, the "spiritual path" which is supposed to get us there is definitely more undefined, more apparently illusory and maybe even a bit unfair (as far as moral people go) than the pursuit of material satisfaction. At least when you have your material things you can look at them and touch them and say, "Look, I have all this money and big houses." And if you are following moral laws you can say, "Look, I am generous, I do not sin, I try to do exactly what God wants me to, I know I am going to Heaven when I die." But what do you have when you have something which can only be described through parables?

I sympathize with the woman in Yeshua' parable, the one who lost a coin and then had to clean the whole house to find it again (Luke 15:9). Was it just that the house was so messy that she had no idea where the coin was? Or is he saying that, in order to find this lost "something," we are going to have to turn everything in our lives upside down? I know from experience that everything in my life was turned upside down a number of times before I got a real sense of what I was looking for.

Most of you will be familiar with the Quest for the Holy Grail. It seems a most silly thing to be doing. Nobody knew what the Grail was. Yet all these knights in shining armour kept galloping around the countryside looking everywhere for it -- looking for something which had no definition.

Yet, if that is not mysterious enough, unlike the Grail knights, Yeshua said you did not have to be morally perfect to enter the Kingdom. In fact, as we have seen, he had many "prostitutes and sinners" as followers, much to the dismay of the holy people of his day. This inclusion of "prostitutes and sinners" is emphasized over and over in the Gospels. And lest the educated think that they were the only ones able to enter, Yeshua said that you have to become like a little child to enter this Kingdom.

Grails, lost coins, pearls of great price, prostitutes, children? How can you find a common meaning in all of these?

I may say to you that the secret is waiting for you, in the dark corners of yourselves, but that does not help you much, as it didn't help me much until I had more specific instructions. How do you look within? Mostly it's just guts in there! And if I say that you have to look in your "consciousness" or your "mind," you might be inclined to ask, "Is there anything more to consciousness than DNA and brain function? Why even bother looking there?"

I know about this search. I spent years looking everywhere, cleaning every nook and cranny of my life. It is not obvious, and it is not easy to find.

Although I know now that the Kingdom of God is not about death, it is related to death in some subtle ways. When I died, I certainly got a view of another world, one which might be considered the realm where God rules – although I found that God rules everywhere, so death couldn't be what I was looking for. Still, during the Death Experience I did meet Yeshua again, so I know he had gone to prepare a place where I could be with him when the time came, as he said he would. At least that part of the puzzle seemed to fit.

But remember, the description of my death which follows here is not itself a description of the Kingdom of God. It is only a story for you. It was my death. It does not take you closer to the Kingdom of God in yourself. Most of you have not had Near Death Experiences, and even for those of you who have had one or two, mine is just a story. So, for now, treat it as another story, like the parables, which point to the possibility of another "Kingdom." Add it to the other stories we are collecting here. Listen and think and see if it forms part of a pattern of what this Kingdom of God might be.

If you are getting the sense that this is a mystery story, you are right. Nothing on this spiritual path is obvious. That is why, in Zen Buddhism, the master gives the student a *Koan* to solve, a riddle which seems to have no answer – something like, "What is the sound of one hand clapping?" The student works at solving the *Koan* until it becomes so frustrating that suddenly the meaning comes. All of these parables and stories are Koans. Hopefully, as we go further, they will begin to make a kind of sense which is not at all logical. In fact, part of what we are doing here is trying to get beyond logic to another way of seeing. You can not talk about the Kingdom of God in purely logical, materialist terms. It involves a different kind of perception.

Ironically, it was after coming back from my death, after a long search in the literature and philosophy of different countries, after looking in many of the religious traditions of the world for this precious "something" -- it was only when I was forced to stop and look within my physical body that I actually began to experience something of this Kingdom of God. But even that is a mystery at this point. How can you look in your physical body for the spiritual realms? Where is the salt and yeast in a human body?

I do not promise that this is going to be easy. Everyone says, "Read my self-help book. The solution to your problems is easy. Just follow these five steps and you are there. I will manipulate your energy a bit and you will be fine." Many people have spoken to me of their frustration after reading these books which promise to solve all their problems in a jiffy, or after going to workshops which are going to magically open their spiritual nature in a weekend. "Am I just dumb?" they complain. "They make it sound so simple, but I can not seem to understand, deep within me, how to change my life."

It is not easy, even if that sells books. No, it's hard, as most of you have found out already. Finding meaning in today's world is far from easy. And it never has been. Two thousand years ago Yeshua was faced with the same problem and his response is the same as mine will have to be. He said, "Enter by the narrow gate; for wide is the gate and broad is the way that leads to destruction, and there are many who go in by it. Because narrow is the gate and difficult is the way which leads to life, and there are few who find it" (Matt 7:13-14).

The other road, the one which finally leads only to more meaninglessness, is the easy one. This one that we are on, the one that leads to the inner realms of God, is the narrow, difficult road that only a few people find. This is the road less travelled. Taking this road requires courage and endurance. Taking this road makes all the difference.

It took a long time for me to find the narrow path. I tried so many others. But it was finally through the practice of what I came to know as the Prayer of Silence that I began to rediscover this inner Light which I had lost. And notice, you are not trying to find this inner Kingdom for the first time – you are trying to remember how to get there, because you came from there in the first place.

Let's take this a little further and be honest with each other.

When you have a chance to talk to people about their deepest longings, as I have in many years of teaching and counselling, you discover that for so many of them, the deepest, secret desire is "to know God." Even those who claim to be atheists have told me of the longing which is deeper that the ideas which led to their atheism. If only they could believe, they say, but the evidence of their senses and their rational theories tell them there is no God. But still, knowing

God, finding the Grail, moving beyond the sense of tremendous cosmic loss or the fear of being alone in the infinite universe -- these things are deepest in us. We know, in some hidden part of ourselves, that there is another way of living than the one which is "of this world."

***

Gnosis and the Knowledge of God

Some languages have special words for the distinctions we are making and for the contrasts and longing we are talking about here. I have found Greek concepts helpful in explaining more clearly a couple of distinctions in meaning which will help us understand. The Greeks had two words for "knowing," one of which leads to the Inner Kingdom. In the process of knowing, they said, there are two distinct mental processes -- *episteme* and *gnosis*.

In *episteme* we know *about* something, we have "epistemological" knowledge -- and religious doctrines and dogmas, philosophical speculations and scientific theories of all sorts, belong here. Doctrines, beliefs and theories are ideas which we formulate on the basis of the evidence available to us. Each religious group, each scientific group, each political group formulates its own list of theories or beliefs which it feels will somehow make sense of its world. It is very easy to fight about doctrines and theories and to get caught in the struggle to try to make "my" ideas dominant over those of others because they are "right." In this kind of epistemological knowing we can even begin to think that people who don't have the same ideas as we do, are crazy or stupid or are even going to Hell. We might even feel justified in killing them, blowing them up, torturing them, because they are obviously sinners or infidels or people of error.

If we want to know God epistemologically, we might go to university or a theological college and learn about God as a theologian or philosopher does, with all the theory and theology. But again, we can learn all the theories about God, as we might learn about all the qualities of a fictitious beast or all the baseball scores of the past ten years, without having any fulfilling sense that our knowledge actually makes a difference. This kind of knowing, the Greek philosophers said, did not help to fill the void within us. Intellectual knowledge is fine for a while and often it is extremely useful or valuable. But then the inner emptiness returns, because doctrine, argument and theoretical knowledge about God do not include any sense of the reality of God's Presence. We are human. We want something we can feel, not just ideas in the head. In times of difficulty, when we feel alone in the universe, theoretical knowledge seems like nothing more than a cruel irrelevancy.

For the Greeks, the other kind of knowing was called *gnosis*. *Gnosis* is how I know my wife and my children and my friends. It is a relationship. It is not theoretical. There is an actual feeling of connection in *gnosis*. When we apply that to our knowledge of God, in *gnosis* we can know God, as Moses, Elijah and Yeshua did. In *gnosis*, God is encountered as a friend, as a "still, small voice," as "Abba, Father," as an enfolding Presence.

But we can go further. In human relationships, the other person is always outside us, independent and separate, no matter how close. They are always the "other," because they inhabit their own skin. In the *"Gnosis of God"* there is something much deeper than any relationship we can have with a person. In this kind of *Gnosis*, of knowing, it is claimed that we can experience God actually within us.

Does this sound familiar? "The Kingdom of God is within," Yeshua says. The realm where you will find God is within. It is like salt or yeast which is baked right into the bread. There is no separation, no separateness in this kind of "knowledge of God." In *Gnosis* there is no other.

It is this *Gnosis*, this inseparable connection to the Divine within, which is central to our experience of God in the Prayer of Silence. This is the experience that children often have. This is the experience which the "prostitutes and sinners" of Yeshua's day found so appealing, because he took them beyond the laws of his native Judaism which condemned them, to an inner awareness of divine love where they did not feel excluded and apart. They knew they belonged to the God Yeshua told them about.

"Gnosticism," the claim that we can actually know God in the secret, inner room of our lives, has gotten a lot of bad press in most churches recently. However, if book sales are any indication, many people are interested in the Gnostic traditions at the present time. The *Gnosticism* which is condemned by many, however, is not what we are talking about here.

Many of the ancient Gnostic groups taught that the universe was divided between the forces of good and evil, often personified as a battle between God and the Devil/Satan, between spirit (good) and flesh (evil) or between Heaven and earth/Hell. As you can see, most present day Christian and Muslim groups would have to be categorized as Gnostic in the ancient sense because they believe in these "dualistic" ideas.

Even though we are talking about being "dwellers in two worlds" in the Prayer of Silence, Yeshua did not teach that the universe was split in two. In fact, he tried to make people aware of the oneness of God and us and the world. "If you want to see God," he implied often, "look at the grass and the flowers and the birds and the wheat and the wind and the things of nature which have come from God. There is no separation between the world and God, only between human beings and God, and that separation is only an illusion because the Kingdom of God is actually within you."

Gnosis emphasizes that we must begin to discover in ourselves an inner knowing of God. We begin to take seriously Yeshua's statement that "the Kingdom of God is within you." We start to move our attention from the externals of the world or the intellectual claims of theory or doctrine, to the Kingdom which is within. We move beyond doctrine and theory to an actual sense of God's Presence within and around us.

***

Putting away childish things

When I look back over my life, I realize that I have, like many others, been involved in this search for the Kingdom of God since childhood. Or, more accurately, it was after my childhood years that I began to search because, as a child, I had a sense of the Presence of God which many children have. Most children do not need to search.

Perhaps that is why Yeshua said, when the disciples tried to send the children away, "Let the little children come to Me, and do not forbid them; for of such is the kingdom of heaven." (Matt 19:14). It is ironic that St. Paul says almost the opposite to what Yeshua says here when he writes in his letter to the Corinthians, "When I was a child, I spoke as a child, I understood as a child, I thought as a child; but when I became a man, I put away childish things" (I Cor. 13:11).

From as far back as I can remember, I wanted to know God. Because this book is a result of my lifelong search for this knowing, it might be helpful if I gave you a short account of some of the highlights of that quest. You might even find some parallels with your own experience which could be of help in clarifying your search.

As a child, growing up in a hot and dusty part of central India, I especially liked the story of God talking to the young Samuel in the Temple. I could imagine Samuel, a small boy like me, walking around the brick pillars of the church in the city of Ujjain where we lived. His mother could have been any one of the many village women going by on oxcarts on the dusty road out front. The idea that God could actually talk to me, as to Samuel, seemed very possible, very much part of that everyday, hot, dusty landscape.

When I was introduced to the other stories, of Moses and Elijah and Yeshua, I found they reinforced that sense that an intimate friendship with God was possible. Moses used to meet with God in a tent on the edge of the encampment of the Hebrews. It was called the Tent of Meeting, and they could discuss whatever they wanted there, Moses even complaining to God about the hard job he had to do.

I seemed to collect these stories in a special part of my memory. Elijah was another. After his contest with King Ahab and Queen Jezebel, he fled into the wilderness. While he was hiding in a cave, a great wind storm, a fire and an earthquake came past the mouth of the cave. But, we are told, God was in none of those. Then Elijah heard a "still small voice" (I Kings 19:12). When he heard this familiar voice, he knew that he was in God's presence, so he covered his head and stood at the mouth of the cave to listen.

We lived part of the year in central India and part in the mountains of north India, the landscape where, for millennia, people had sought God in the caves and valleys of this land of eternal snow. I could easily sense that God was in the gentle sighing of the wind through the branches of the giant deodar trees, in the stillness of a glade in the woods or at the rocky source of the Ganges River with permanent, snow covered mountains soaring 25,000 feet into the sky. In fact, the whole of the landscape seemed to be alive with the potential presence of God. And I knew, even as a child, why people would spend their lives there, seeking God's presence.

At the age of about five or six I had an experience which confirmed this perception. I was standing on a path in the mountains. Through the space between two other mountains below me, I could see just a small part of the Dun Valley even farther below. Suddenly, it was as if I rose out of my body, moving not only above my child's body, but also into the past, before I had been born.

I had the sense that the Dun Valley was like the valley of time. I was looking at myself looking at it and remembering a time before I was born when I had looked down on time and decided to be born at a particular point in history. I knew I could have been born up the valley to the right, sometime in the future, or even down the valley to the left, sometime in the past. But for some unknown reason I had chosen now instead. It was a wonderful perception and seemed to open up the whole landscape of time and life to mystery and possibility. I did not know why I had been born now, but I knew I had chosen. Later in life, I could sympathize with Jeremiah who said that he knew God had chosen him for a particular job before he was even in the womb. I knew many people had been chosen in the same way.

Then I came back to my little body, very excited. But when I told my story to others, they seemed to have no idea what I was talking about and ridiculed or condemned the implications of my vision. So I stopped talking about it, but kept it as one of the mysteries of childhood I had to figure out later in life.

Since then I have discovered that many young children remember these things, times before they were born, lives they have lived elsewhere. But then they usually forget because adults tell them it is all nonsense and they put away these precious childish things. Had I come into the world from some kind of Kingdom of God, I wondered for many years?

I grew up in a Christian home, with devout parents, so I knew that Christianity was central to my life. But I knew that there were a lot of other people in India who devoted their lives to God, and they were not of my faith.

On the streets of the cities, on the country paths or in the sacred city of Ujjain you could always find Hindu "holy men", "*sadhus*, who had left everything to find God. There were the Jains in white robes, sweeping their paths so that they would not inadvertently kill any living creatures as they walked by. There was the old Muslim man who used to sit regularly by the side of the road with the Koran on a reading stand, performing his devotions. The Tibetan Buddhists used to come to Mussoorie, where we went to school, to trade goods and to put up their prayer flags on what we called Prayer Flag Hill. I was even able as a youth, in 1959, to see the Dalai Lama, also a young man at that time, who had just fled the Chinese invasion and had settled not far from where we lived. And there were the devout village Christians, coming to the communion service in spotless clothing or singing songs of devotion to the beat of a drum in an aboriginal village late in the night near the city of Ratlam where we lived for a while.

All these seemed in my child's imagination like the Old Testament prophets, wandering over the land, communing with God. It was hard for a child to make distinctions of doctrine when there was so much obvious devotion to the Divine in all these people.

Yeshua could easily have been any one of these. He wandered like the *sadhus* and had no fixed address. He was God-intoxicated, going into the wilderness to commune with Abba, Father. He had obviously devoted his life to God and had discovered, in his wanderings, that anyone could come to God in the same way. "We are all children of the Father," he said. No one was excluded. The God who he spoke about was like a father who loved his children, even when they went astray. His was an accepting God, one who did not condemn. You could talk lightly to this kind of God as even a child would talk to his parents.

Like many children, I did talk to God and to Yeshua when I was young, and found great comfort in that. But unfortunately, like most children, I assumed that this kind of talk was what children did and that, when I grew up, the adults would be able to tell me the real way to talk to God. Surely, I reasoned in my child's mind, the adults must know even more of how to do this. All those ministers and missionaries must be really intimate with God, like Moses was.

So, gradually, I began to think that I would "put away my childish things" and develop a more "mature" way of relating to God.

It was a great disappointment to find that most of the adults didn't know how to establish that kind of relationship. They spoke of God being in Heaven, "above" us somehow, far away from us, outside of our world. We were going to go to that Heaven to "be with God" when we died.

Then, when I was old enough to go to school, some of the visiting preachers began to portray God as really quite frightening. If we did not repent of our "sins," whatever those were, we would end up in a burning place called Hell. One of my friends from a conservative church told me in graphic detail what Hell was like. So I began to get very frightened. I would confess any little wrong I did as soon as I did it, because I was afraid God would send me to this everlasting torment. What if I fell down one of the ever-present cliffs which yawned beneath us on the path to school every day, after committing a sin without confessing? What if I committed "the sin against the Holy Spirit," when no one knew what it was? What if I didn't even know I had sinned?

This was a completely different god [I cannot use a capital G for this god] than the one I had encountered as a child. Here was a frightening judge, someone capable of intentionally inflicting infinite torture even on little children. This really didn't seem like the kind of person you would want to get too close to -- certainly not the loving Father Yeshua talked about. In fact, it might be just as well to stay as far away from this kind of god as possible. It was best to let him stay up at the holy end of the church and keep him from getting on too intimate terms with your everyday activities.

As I grew older, this god became even more difficult and even more distant, and the fear did not completely disappear for many years. I became aware of the terrible, helpless, lonely terror which lies at the heart of most believers in the monotheistic religions – that fear of being unworthy, of deserving infinite torture even though we did not ask to be created. This doctrine of Hell and damnation and infinite suffering, imposed by a god who could not be placated except by the human sacrifice of his own son, made a mockery of all the teaching of Yeshua. What kind of "loving Father" would do that kind of thing? Yet that is what so many preachers and their followers teach with full conviction.

The universe began to take on the colouring of madness, a place where it was impossible to escape fear and torture and abject terror – a place where love and joy and peace became ever more distant and almost hopeless goals. I saw this terror in so many people around me, in the children who huddled and talked in hushed voices about their own fears. How was I to escape what could not be escaped?

Only later did I discover that Hell and Satan/Shaitan came originally from the ancient Zoroastrian belief in two gods, Ahura Mazda and Ahriman, who ruled the destiny of humanity. That belief had lived on to torture countless billions of believers in many religions. But for me, growing up in a boarding school, far from the security of home and parents, with a war threatening between India and China not far to the north of us, the universe was becoming a very frightening place where not even God could be trusted.

I have since concluded that this message of fear is a form of deep child abuse which should be named what it is and should be abandoned as a way of trying to "frighten people into salvation," as I have heard it called by the people who preach it.

It took a long time to get over this inner terror at the idea that there was no escape from infinite torture – that the deity which I had known as loving turned out to be a psychopath, at least in the eyes of so many of the adults I trusted. In fact, for many years, I even found it difficult to use the name, "God," because of the fear that was associated with it.

I had to find a way around this fear and did so by adopting another name for God. Indian Christians called God "Ishwar" (pronounced Eesh-waar). It was the Hindu name for the personal aspect of God and I was able to speak to Ishwar in prayer when I found it difficult to speak to the deity which the evangelists had turned into a source of inner terror. I was finally able to overcome this terror and was able to start talking to "God" again, but it took a long time and much inner work. I shudder to think how many people are trapped in that same fear now. If you are one of those, I hope you will be free of it once you learn to practice the Prayer of Silence exercises which are designed to overcome just such fears.

But before I had a chance to resolve those fears, I became more "mature." I was introduced at university, where I went to study for the Christian ministry, to complicated theologies which made it seem as if you could only really know God once you had studied a great deal. God became more of an idea in the brain or a complex set of intellectual propositions. Of course, most theologies asserted that God had somehow "come in Jesus," (whatever that meant) and God's humanity was manifest in this way, but that was also only theory and doctrine. The quarrels over the nature of that "incarnation" had led to the splits of churches and religions, to war and all manner of bickering and evil, murder and suicide.

The "advanced theologians," learning from materialist psychology, determined that none of the miracles attributed to Jesus actually happened and, because of misdating of ancient ruins and inscriptions during the 19th century, scholars even claimed that nothing in the Bible actually happened, that it was all made up.

(To understand the nature of this mis-dating, read David Rohl's books, *A Test of Time: the Bible -- from Myth to History* as well as *From Eden to Exile: the Epic History of the People of the Bible*. He presents archaeological evidence which suggests that the Bible is actually very accurate in its description of events, once the dates assigned to the Egyptian dynasties are adjusted according to modern scientific observation methods. All other events in Middle Eastern chronology are always coordinated with the Egyptian dates to establish time lines for ancient history.)

And then, as I grew even older, I discovered that most of the adults seemed to feel deserted by God or to feel that God didn't even exist.

So, like many others, I lost that child-like trust and entered the spiritual wasteland of adulthood. God was an abstraction. Yeshua was someone who had come and gone many years before. I persuaded myself that there were important messages in the Bible, but they did not seem to get to the heart of the spiritual longing I felt, nor did they seem to speak to the longing of many of my contemporaries. It was as if the stories of Moses and Elijah and Samuel were just teasing in a cruel sort of way. If they could have that close relationship with God, why couldn't I? Why couldn't others? Were the stories merely myths arising from wishful thinking, as many writers asserted? Was God just a way for us to deal with the anxiety of death, as Freud claimed?

And how could I get beyond the fear monger churches or religions, the Hell-fire preachers who portrayed God as an extremely cruel judge, as a psychopath who tortured people who hadn't even asked to be born? How could I take part in that kind of belief and its obvious gross injustice as a minister preaching that kind of thing? So, like many people in my generation, in all generations, I struggled and railed and fought, looking for answers.

But something in me couldn't let go of this "God thing." Like many millions of people, in spite of my disappointment, the greater longing resulted in a life-long search for the kind of intimate relationship with God which the biblical text suggested was possible. Was it?

Maybe it was merely wishful thinking. Maybe there wasn't anything there to find. Maybe we only had this world in which to live, and this world had no meaning. But this longing for the Divine was very deep and came from the most important sub-strata of my being -- maybe even from the centre of my being. So, through all the vicissitudes of life, I followed this urge to find God, even if it was going to lead only to emptiness.

Like many others, I caught glimpses of a divine presence from time to time. Especially in nature there seemed to be something which could be called "God." Whether it was in the soft breeze by a prairie field in the evening stillness of western Canada, or a sense of actual Presence walking in a valley in the Rocky Mountains, at least there seemed to be the potential of something real beyond the theories and the fears.

Little did I expect the insight and understanding -- the pure bliss and love and joy, sometimes -- that would eventually arise from that search. Nor did I anticipate the deep struggle with the self which accompanied and preceded those insights.

It is out of this struggle and its fruits that the present guide to meditation has grown.

***

Entering the kingdom of death

In most religions, death is considered the final enemy, the final kingdom of fear. Many Christian theologians even teach that Jesus somehow defeated the final enemy, death, the final realm where Satan rules. Yet I found it completely different from what the theologians teach. I found that even death is an expression of God's love and is not something to fear. It is certainly not the realm where Satan rules!

Everything changed in 1966 when I died. In June of that year, in the city of Regina, Saskatchewan, Canada, I fell down an unmarked 37 foot (11 meter) piling shaft on a construction site. When my heels finally hit bottom, the shock drove like a pile driver up through my back, crushing one of my vertebrae to half its size and badly fracturing two others. The tremendous shock tore my internal organs out of place. After rescue and a rush to the hospital, I spent a couple of days in and out of consciousness. Then I died.

It is important to pay close attention to this account. It will give you an experiential basis for your initiation into the other world in which you will start to live shortly. I will describe the Near Death Experience in detail, because there are many elements in it which will tell you a great deal about your own consciousness, as it taught me many things about mine. I will refer to it often in the pages ahead because it will clarify much of what you are trying to achieve.

Dying is amazing. It takes us past the limits of body and senses into a whole new world – you might even say, into a new kingdom.

A couple of nights after the accident, my physical system went into distress. The nurses came running and called the emergency team but, as they worked on me, I sensed that my body was somehow falling apart. Then I lost objective consciousness of the body and the hospital, but discovered, to my surprise, that I was not unconscious.

Once the body awareness was gone, I became aware of a different reality. The story which has changed everything began when the hospital vanished.

After I "came back," one of the nurses told me, "We thought we had lost you. We did everything we could to bring you back, and then suddenly, when we had just about given up, there you were again."

I had survived, but it was a very different me who returned. When I came back, I carried with me a mystery that would take my whole life to unravel.

The first indication that I was dying was that I found myself looking at the body, which I had thought was me, from somewhere just above my left shoulder. I seemed to be both apart from and yet still in the body.

I could sense that underlying, surrounding and interpenetrating this physical system which was breaking down, was another organizing principle. It was a living, interconnected network which was more subtle than the body, organs, emotions and ideas which are the most obvious features of our nature. I realized that my life in the body had depended on two, parallel worlds working in harmony.

There was the physical system of organs and tissues, which was now falling apart. But this physical system seemed to be a manifestation of a more subtle energy network which was itself a link between my "consciousness" (from which I was looking and which I later called the Watcher) and the physical body. I, the Watcher, was somehow linked through this energy network with the more dense body network.

This underlying, organizational network was separating from the body.

It is hard to explain, but I became aware concurrently of several levels of what I had thought was simply "me." I was conscious of every cell in my body all at the same time. I was also conscious that all my memories somehow existed in the cells of both the body and brain, as well as in the "mind," and that I was watching all of this from the point just above my left shoulder. It became obvious that there were quite a number of levels and systems involved just in the memories I was harvesting.

I was aware that there was a life force holding the cells together, like glue or a magnetic field, but I could also feel that this life force, which was holding all the elements of the physical systems in place, was coming apart. It was as if I was standing back, looking from a place outside the body, yet I was still connected with all the processes taking place in the body.

And, more importantly, I became aware that the centre of consciousness from which I observed all of this complex activity, the "Watcher" which I found myself to be in a sense more fundamental than any other aspect of my whole, living, interconnected being, was much more real than anything else in the body.

At the time of my "death" I was tremendously alive. And I sensed that this observing, yet extremely active aspect of the whole of what had been "Bruce," was somehow the source from which everything else manifested and functioned.

However, this observing source of my life was also the way I was connected to the "spiritual," non-physical aspects of the universe. It was through this "Watcher" that I was able to talk to Jesus shortly after my "death." It was only later, when I discovered its function in meditation, that I called this aspect of the self "the Watcher."

We will come back to this Watcher many times in what follows here because I have found a way of making you aware of this aspect of yourself very quickly in meditation. It is from this perspective that you can learn the deepest realities in your world. The Watcher can change your whole life once you learn how it works.

As I watched the process of my own death, I thought, with great interest, "Wow, this is what it is like to die." This awareness was a strange, new way of knowing. It wasn't brain knowledge, since I was outside of the brain, observing from just above my left shoulder. It was not body knowledge, either, because the body was coming apart. It was a different, non-rational, non-brain, totally inclusive kind of knowing that, "This is what it's like to die." It was as if I had entered suddenly into *Gnosis*.

Here was a tremendous discovery. There was no fear, no doubt and no pain -- just a sense of matter-of-factness. What I thought of as this "new me," (although it was actually the spiritual origins of my life in the body) this Watcher, watched the process of withdrawal with great interest, but at the same time was actively involved in the withdrawal. It was as if this new me was gathering up all the impressions of the life that had been, impressions which were somehow stored in every cell in that body and brain. I knew somehow (because I seemed to be connected with a whole level of meaning "above" the body through the Watcher) that the life of the person I was leaving was ending, that the purpose of that life had been fulfilled, and I was now "harvesting" all that it had experienced.

There was no sense of loss. I knew at that moment that the ego, the Bruce personality to which I had been attached in my short life, was fleeting, almost illusory. But I also knew that something else, some other aspect of my being, was real in a way that the body and its life could never be. Words, ego, fear, self-defence, even self itself, didn't seem to matter at that point. The old body and sense-based ideas were left behind and I was focussed in a completely different state of being where things were known directly and instantly and with a sense of wholeness.

Finally, I completed the separation. Once all the memories had been "harvested," I willed the life-force to withdraw from the cells. The intermediate network no longer had to maintain the pattern of the life that had been "Bruce," and the body could be left behind in the hospital.

Then the scene changed. I had moved from the body, from the hospital, to a "place" which was not a place at all, but more like a transitional state of being. The landscape, if you could call it that, was a light, self-luminous grey, almost like clouds but more flat and extending into the distance. I sensed that, in this landscape, distance was time, and the farther I looked in front of me, the farther back in time I looked.

To the left, going gently upward, was the tunnel of light which has become so familiar in Near Death Experience accounts. The tunnel seemed to be related, not to movement in space, but to movement between states of being. If I went up that amazingly attractive tunnel of light, to the love I could sense was there, I would move into a different aspect of spiritual consciousness, not into a different place. I seemed to be in a world, not of time and space, but of different dimensions of awareness and being. I also knew that I would not want to return to the life of the body if I went through that tunnel.

I had no idea at the time that other people had these experiences. It was not until 1975, almost ten years later, that the first book was published on Near Death Experiences.

There was the tunnel of light, a bit to my left, and I knew that it was possible for me to go there if I wanted. But I was also aware of three men in vaguely Middle Eastern dress, silhouetted against the tunnel of light and the time landscape. Before I could decide to go up the tunnel of light, I had to discuss a number of things with them. We discussed a "project" (which I will explain in a moment).

I recognized these men immediately, and we had a long conversation. They seemed to be old friends, and it seemed like we had worked together before. I haven't told many people who they were for most of the years since then, and was even reluctant to admit it to myself when I came back to life, it seemed so impossible. When telling of my Near Death Experience I always said, "I spoke with three men," leaving them nameless. But, as I have already described in *The Thomas Book*, it was Yeshua, Elijah and Moses who stood there, however unlikely that may seem, and however unlikely the parallels with Yeshua's experience on the Mount of Transfiguration may seem. In fact, there seemed to be a continuation from that scene on the mountain, in this experience in the realms of death. The project was a continuation of what they had discussed there, two thousand years earlier.

Why these three? I later came to realize that what I have learned and am now teaching is part of a spiritual tradition stretching back through time, through the Judeo-Christian past reflected in the Bible, back into the Egyptian mysteries from which Moses learned, and even earlier than that. Jewish and Christian researchers have known for a long time that there is a tradition of spirituality underlying many of the stories in the Bible. They know that there were "schools of the prophets" which taught some form of spirituality.

There seemed to be major phases of the development of these "schools." Moses introduced the Hebrew slaves of Egypt to the initial stages of the teaching, to the laws and sense of order involved in the worship of one God. Elijah taught many prophets in his "school of the prophets" and preserved the message even when it was close to extinction at the hands of King Ahab and Queen Jezebel. The community which produced the Dead Sea Scrolls was a continuation of Elijah's school. Yeshua spread the message internationally and invited even the outcasts of society to learn of the inner love of God.

There are ancient accounts of the fall of souls into materiality, their becoming trapped there and a continuing attempt made to teach souls that they can be liberated from their imprisonment in the world of the flesh, of cause and effect and suffering. Historically, there have been several lines of tradition where teachers have been born to try to teach souls of their potential to live in spirit rather than in the prison of materiality. Although these traditions are all related to each other in their basic tenets, they also have geographical centres which delineate distinct traditions. These seem to centre on India/Europe (Sanskrit source religions), on China, on North and South America and on the Mediterranean/Africa. There are also the shamanic traditions of most aboriginal peoples. There has been much carryover from one tradition to another because they all have the same aims of liberating people from the negative, materialist, divisive forces in the world.

What I was drawn into in my Near Death Experience, and what I was taught later, seems to be an expression of the living biblical tradition, an extension of the Mediterranean/African (Egyptian) tradition reflected in the experience of the prophets and of Yeshua. This spiritual tradition and its practices (which are independent of the legalist traditions of the Bible) are not spelled out clearly in the Bible because most of the writers of the Bible were either not initiated into this tradition, or had promised during their initiation not to reveal its secrets. We have only brief glimpses of it in the present biblical text.

It is interesting for me to read the biblical accounts of this spiritual tradition in the light of my Death Experience. Much of what I explain about the Prayer of Silence will be illustrated with reference to the hints about that hidden biblical tradition. Yeshua's teachings about the inner Kingdom of God are part of the tradition, and the "project" which we four discussed had to do partly with conveying that tradition more openly to any who were interested. This book is part of the project. *The Thomas Book* was the other major, foundation document I had to write.

In the Near Death Experience, Yeshua was to my left, facing me, and closest to me. I could see the tunnel of light over his right shoulder. Elijah was a bit to my right and farther back. Moses stood almost in the middle, seemingly between Yeshua and Elijah, but even farther back, receding in time from me. I had the odd sense of communicating through time rather than through space.

We talked about a number of issues, including the project I have just spoken of, for what seemed to be quite a while. I have found it frustrating, since coming back, that the details of our conversation have been vague, as if a screen was put up in my mind to keep me from remembering. Perhaps I could not accept in my conscious mind what I had seen then. Or, more likely, forgetfulness had descended so that I would have to work to recover what we had talked about. I had to enter deep into the mysteries of spiritual consciousness through meditation so that I could later teach those things. In the process, I would discover things about our spiritual nature and about the world which can only come through a life of meditation and inner exploration.

For many years after I returned to life, I refused to acknowledge what I knew, because it was such a shock to all my conscious pre-conceptions. My religious upbringing, my education in the materialist West, my ideas about death and life beyond death were all put sorely to the test. But, however much I ignored it, the memory of this event was always there in the background, pushing me along in an extended search for answers.

Although I didn't remember the details, I did remember that we talked about why I had been in that body lying back there in the hospital and why I had chosen to come into life now -- which seemed to refer to the experience I had as a child in India, looking at the Valley of Time. But now the body was smashed up badly and didn't work anymore. I, the Self which somehow transcended the little ego self, had withdrawn from that body and had even taken away the force which held it in life. Bruce had died and we had to decide what to do now.

I have often wondered if the "accident" was supposed to be the end of my life or if it had been much worse than had been intended. I now realize that my life was complete when I died in 1966. I could have chosen to stay in the realms of spirit. But in choosing to return to the body, I essentially began another life. It was as if I was incarnated again, perhaps to experience vividly the whole process of reincarnation. Later, in 1991, I died another kind of death – the death of the brain and its memories -- and started another life, so that I have lived three lives in this one life.

At the end of our discussion, Yeshua said to me, "You can come now, or you can go back." By this he meant, I could come up into the Light or I could go back into the body.

It was a difficult decision. I hesitated for a while, thinking about all its implications. The Light was tremendously attractive and the body back on that narrow Stryker Frame was not even ready to support life. I knew my hesitation arose from the conflict of being attracted to the Light but also of wanting to complete the project for which I had been in that broken body.

Yeshua said, cautioning me before I made my decision, "Remember, if you go back into the body, it's pretty badly smashed up. You do not have to return. We can do this another way."

I replied, "Well, yeah, OK," in a noncommittal way.

And I thought about it a little bit more, about what needed to be done, about the project we were involved in and that Bruce had been planning to be part of, and I said, "I've got a few things I need to do still. I think I'll go back." I also remembered that I had been engaged to a young woman just days before the accident and that she was somehow involved in this whole project. I didn't realize that two children were waiting to come into our family. I had many things to return to.

Then Yeshua cautioned me again, "Remember, the body is badly smashed up. It will take a lot of effort to get it going again. You do not have to go back. We can do things in another way."

But I said, "That's all right. I'll go back."

Then the third time Yeshua warned me, almost severely this time, "You do not have to do this. Remember, the old machine is really badly smashed up. It will take a lot of work to get it going again. You don't have to go back. We can do this some other way." And I knew I would be taking on a very big task if I decided to go back to the body.

But I also knew I had to return and I said, "That's alright. I have to go back."

There was no transition, no farewell. Instantly, I was back near the body but not in it. In fact, the body was not ready to support life, so I couldn't get in. It had died. But I also couldn't leave. I was now in the position of not having a body to go to, but not being able to return to the spiritual state I was in before.

I found myself in that earlier position of observing the body as the Watcher, when I had watched the "glue" let go. But this time I knew I couldn't just jump back into the body, since it wasn't ready. It came to me that I actually had to will the cells back together again. If I could reverse the process I had been involved in earlier, where I had withdrawn the memories and the life force from all the cells, then I realized I could reactivate the body and make it work.

I also realized that it was somehow my "spiritual will" which would make it possible to "get the old machine going again," and I had to assert that will with all my spiritual force. Even in the Near Death Experience I knew that this must have been a variation of what Yeshua had to do to get back into the body after his death. There were certain things I had to learn about life and death in order to fulfil my work, and these things had to be learned first hand, not through abstract teachings.

Through this experience, I learned that what I call the Watcher aspect of my spiritual consciousness was very powerful -- it was not just an observer of events. It was a centre of spiritual awareness but also a centre of spiritual will, creativity and power, as well as the centre of my spiritual being.

Once I realized what I had to do, I could feel the reintegration process starting in the whole body. It was as if I was providing a conscious, magnetic field, the supportive network I had sensed earlier, in which all the elements of what we know as human life could begin to function again. But this was much more subtle and purposeful than merely a magnetic field. This seemed to be a Spiritual Field, a Life Energy Field which carried in itself all the patterns which make human life possible. The Watcher was capable of doing all of this.

When I woke, I was back in the body again, back in the limiting, physical shell, immobilised on a Stryker Frame in the hospital, as if to emphasize the limits of the body. That was it. I had gone through the short time which changed my life.

That was my initiation into the mysteries of human consciousness.

My real training began after the initiation. I did not just have to get the old machine going again. I had to discover, deep in my own soul, what the Death Experience implied about human consciousness, and then how that awareness could be presented so that other people could use the new awareness to speed up their own spiritual growth. This was to be part of the project we four had discussed.

I was faced with two major tasks.

First, I knew there was something very wrong with the Gospel stories in the Bible. I had to find out what that mystery was about, and I have done that in a book called *The Thomas Book: Near Death, a Quest and a New Gospel by the Twin Brother of Jesus* (Eloquent Books, 2010).

Second, I knew that human consciousness was very different from what was reflected in most of the modern theories of personality, because most of them are based on the materialist idea that the body and brain produce consciousness. I now knew beyond a doubt that the ancient traditions were true, that consciousness not only produced the body and brain, but could even reactivate a body which had died. Consciousness could exist separate from the body. I had to discover in practical terms how that insight could be put to use by others.

Gradually, over the following years, I was drawn inexorably to a complete change in my understanding of life and how the body is related to consciousness, of how our relationships with others function as reflections of our deep spiritual nature, of how we are related to time and the manifestations of our being in other lives, and of what our relationship to the Divine reality, to God, is all about.

I found that my childhood perceptions of our innate ability to communicate with the central Love and Life and Consciousness of the universe had been substantially correct. Now I had to develop and deepen those perceptions with an exploration of this mysterious person which I had found myself to be -- which I had found all of us to be.

In the Death Experience I had been immersed in what Yeshua calls the Kingdom of God, that spiritual dimension of life to which we all have access if only we know where to find the keys.

I spent a long, painful, frustrating seven months in hospital, sometimes regretting intensely my decision to come back into this broken body, and wondering if I should have taken the other path which was offered. However, I learned the importance of persistence, faith, will and spiritual force. It was only through the use of those that I was finally able to overcome the obstacles. I was finally able to get out of the bed into a wheelchair and then I learned to walk all over again. I went from the hospital to the Rehab Centre where I spent many hours pulling myself along the railings, forcing my body to do things it did not seem to welcome. But, in the process, I learned how much the spiritual will can achieve in putting a broken body back together.

I also learned some very important basic lessons about the nature of consciousness, lessons which will find their way over and over into this book.

First, we are not our bodies, our emotions or the little concerns of the ego. We are something much more profound than we can even imagine in our little ego world, but it was only when I was forced to move beyond ego by the necessity to put the body back together, that I was able to become aware, in small part, of who I was capable of becoming.

Nor are we our brains, ideas or beliefs. Brains and ideas are important for providing instant access to information or rational processes, like a computer, but I and you are not this computer. Our central consciousness, the Watcher, is capable of moving, observing, creating, willing and correcting in ways which lie far beyond any of the usual rational or emotional processes we are familiar with.

The aspect of our being which is primarily responsible for creating and maintaining mind, body and emotions is the Watcher. It is, in a sense, detached from our everyday lives because its nature is not tied to time and place. However, it is also intimately involved in every aspect of our lives, in every cell and memory and feeling. It is active, powerful and creative and it can bring about a complete change in our lives, even putting broken bodies and lives back together.

By the end of this book, if you do the exercises here, you will become aware of many of the potentials of this Watcher aspect of the Self. It is the Divine Centre of our being.

***

I knew, as soon as I got out of the hospital in January of 1967, that I had to get back to university. I had much to learn, to fill in the huge areas of ignorance that the Death Experience had made me aware of.

What was the human experience all about? It was obviously very different from the picture I had before the Death Experience. I had to find a way to solve that mystery. And it could not involve just questions of philosophy and theology, which I had been studying before the accident. This experience obviously related to all of what it is to be human.

I also had to learn of the world and of the traditions by which other people had explained life and death. I had grown up in India, Canada and the United States. I had travelled the Atlantic and Mediterranean, the Suez Canal, the Arabian Sea and Indian Ocean. I had a lot of international contact but I needed to learn of this planet and its people in more depth.

Once I got back to university, I discovered that studying literature gave me an excuse to study everything else, since I found that, in order to appreciate novels and plays and poetry, I also had to know about psychology and philosophy and science, about history and sociology, about religion and culture, about mysticism and spiritual longing, about geography and the relations of countries and races and peoples. If I could teach at university, I could get paid to learn all that as part of my job. And if I could teach the literatures of Africa, Canada, Australia, India, the West Indies and other parts of the world, I had a wonderful excuse to read anything I wanted from anywhere in the world I wanted. So, after a process of gradual realization, I determined to take that route.

I left Regina in 1967, a little over a year after the accident. In another nine years, we were back in Regina again, as if we could not get away. In 1968, Olive (to whom I had become engaged just days before the accident) and I had married in her home in Trinidad in the West Indies. I finished a BA and an MA before a stint of teaching at Acadia University in Nova Scotia. Then we went to Leeds in England, where I completed my PhD in World Literature Written in English, and taught in the School of English. Later, back in Canada, I held a teaching appointment at the University of New Brunswick for a year before accepting a position in the English Department at the University of Regina.

We had come full circle. We were back in the city where I had met Yeshua in death and had decided to try to put the old machine back together again.

I had immersed myself in the study of human creativity and language by studying literature and its social and cultural context from around the world. I had also started a career as a sculptor and a writer and had a deep sense of the roots of creativity in myself. I had studied religious mysticism and mystical writers like William Blake, Patrick White, Emanuel Swedenborg, St. John of the Cross, and many others. All of this gave me a rich background in the profound creative potential of humanity.

But I was still unsatisfied. I had not solved the riddle of what was wrong with the Gospels and I had not found a vital, living understanding of what happened during my Death Experience. To put it in terms we are now familiar with, I had a lot of epistemological knowledge which was essential to my later development, but had not yet discovered *Gnosis*.

I had come to the point in my spiritual education where the comment in the medieval spiritual text, *The Cloud of Unknowing*, was directly applicable to me: "So I say that it is good in due time to give up your intellectual exercises, and to learn to taste something of the love of God in your own spiritual experience" (Penguin Books).

The next stage of my spiritual education was to take me deep into the world of *Gnosis* through an interesting, and often painful route when "the old machine" began to malfunction again. It was through the process of solving those difficulties that this present volume was born. It was also in being thrown back into the life of the Spirit that I met Yeshua again, as in the Death Experience, and that *The Thomas Book*, a gospel from the perspective of the Apostle, Didymos Judas Thomas, was written in a mysterious way which I describe in that book.

By 1971, all that remained from the accident was a slight limp. I had gotten the old machine going again. But when we moved to Leeds in 1972, the pain in my back returned. It grew steadily worse over a number of years. In 1976 we returned to Regina. All that time the pain kept growing. In 1978, the year I started teaching at Luther College, a federated college of the University of Regina, the doctor had prescribed narcotic pain killers to keep me going, and the specialists were trying to fit me for a variety of back braces to ease the pain.

By January of 1979, I could take no more, so the specialists did more tests and found that the bone graft on the spinal fusion had been gradually growing on the inside until it was putting great pressure on the spinal cord. Another few months, they said, and I would be paralysed from the waist down. They did emergency surgery and in another eight months I was back at work, but still with a lot of pain.

Did I have to get the old machine going yet again, I wondered? And how could I do it this time? Wasn't I already doing what I was supposed to be doing with my life? What more was required?

It was at that point, in about 1980, that I was introduced to research that was being done on the medical uses of meditation. At first, I did not accept that the mind could heal the body, in spite of all I had been through. Ironically, I still hadn't realized the importance of the discovery I had made about the power of the Watcher -- I still had to learn about that. I was reluctant to try medical meditation exercises because I really didn't believe they could help. After all, they were all psychological, I reasoned, and my pain was caused by actual, solid, physical damage to nerves. But to my surprise, within a week of starting serious meditative visualization exercises, I had gotten rid of the pain.

This was the beginning of another phase of discovery. My physical survival actually depended on learning the difference between *episteme* and *gnosis* and learning the power of the Watcher, the aspect of consciousness through which *gnosis* is achieved.

If the mind in meditation could get rid of pain and disability, what else could it do? Here was an area of ignorance I had to explore. And to my surprise, it led me right back into the Death Experience of 1966. That experience proved to be pivotal in my spiritual life.

In a strange way, I discovered, meditation and death were connected. Both permit us to free consciousness from the constraints of the body. Both make it possible to discover something of tremendous importance about our spiritual nature. One of the most important exercises we do in this book will illustrate this phenomenon to you in a gentle yet convincing way as you become aware of the Watcher aspect of consciousness.

I began a regular schedule of meditation and read voraciously anything which might give insights into this whole area of experience. During the 1970s and 80s there was a lot of research being done on bio-feedback, meditation and healing, and other aspects of the mind/body interaction. Books were being published on various aspects of Near Death Experiences. However, no one else seemed to have entered into this area of experience in the same way I was being led.

After about a year of regular meditation, I met Yeshua again in my inner being. I was doing my regular meditation when he appeared to my "mind's eye." He welcomed me with a smile, and asked with a great sense of humour,

"Why did it take so long to find your way back here?" Apparently, I had managed to solve a puzzle.

Meditation, I then realized, had brought me back to the same level of consciousness I had been in during the Near Death Experience. I learned a very important lesson: death is not an end -- it is merely a shift of consciousness whereby we can move our awareness in a dramatic way out of our physical body. Meditation is a similar shift of consciousness, except that we are able to return at will to the body, because there is still that vital link which keeps the body functioning. Now that I had found my way back to that state of consciousness, two questions arose: how much could consciousness achieve in this shifted state and, could I teach others to make this shift of consciousness? Was this phenomenon repeatable?

And still there was the nagging question: what was wrong with the Gospels?

I had suppressed much of what went on in our meeting during the Near Death Experience. In 1966 I couldn't believe that I would meet Yeshua, and especially not with Elijah and Moses into the bargain. That seemed just a little too much to take. But now, during the early 1980s, in the regular silence of meditation, I was brought back to the experience of that time. This stage of my learning involved more than just the cultures and literatures of the world: it also involved, through actual experience, discoveries about the deep spiritual nature of humanity.

And here is where *The Thomas Book*, and later, *The Prayer of Silence*, grew as well.

During my meditations I kept a journal, writing down experiences and perceptions as they arose. Yeshua guided me with hints and suggestions during my meditations. Working on his suggestions, I then had to discover the meaning of the hints for my everyday life.

It was a difficult and often painful form of learning. I was instructed, pushed to discover things for myself, then given more hints and sent into the regular world of a university professor -- of teaching, marking essays, counselling, attending meetings and dealing with hundreds of relationships, as well as maintaining a marriage and family -- to learn how the hints applied. I was being taught how my inner being was reflected in my outer life, and how my actions and thoughts and attitudes in that outer life were reflected in my inner life. It was a bit like what you have been doing with your daily review meditations.

From about 1980 to 1991 I continued an intense program of meditation, along with my usual work as a university professor. As part of my research, I was able to travel to conferences and on research and speaking trips to different parts of Canada, Trinidad, England, the US, Malta and India. In the process I had many experiences which furthered my inner search.

I also did a lot of personal counselling of students and members of the community. Word began to spread that I knew of a different way of resolving problems. Friends referred their friends and relatives to me so that a lot of people benefited from the problem solving aspects of the Prayer of Silence in this early stage of my learning.

But the real test of the effectiveness of the Prayer of Silence, as I came to know this method, was yet to come. That is where my advanced spiritual education really began.

In 1991 I got a serious case of viral encephalitis, the inflammation of the lining of the brain. The disease wiped out vast amounts of memory, completely destroyed my personality and brought an end to my teaching career. I could hardly sign my name and had trouble even copying numbers or words. I couldn't recognize people I had known for years. My brain had been badly damaged. Yet again, my life seemed to have come to a complete halt.

However, as I struggled through this new area of darkness, I realized that the Near Death Experience and meditation had both taught me that I was not my body. Now, as I began to put the lessons of the Prayer of Silence into practice in order to recover memory, I discovered a tremendously important lesson --- I was not my brain. That was a hard principle to learn, since my whole career had been based on brain knowledge. But it was also a tremendously important principle to learn, since it made it possible to rebuild my brain and its functions.

After the accident, I had put the body back together using my spiritual will to force the body to work: now I had to put the brain back together using a similar method, but at a much deeper level.

I began the long process of using meditative techniques to put my brain, my memory, my relationships and my life back together. (People who have had brain damage can benefit greatly from the exercises in this book, since they were designed in part to overcome that particular problem.)

I knew from my earlier experience of coming back to an essentially dead body, that when I was able to view myself from the position of the Watcher, I could provide a spiritual network and energy patterns to get the body going again. I discovered I could also rebuild the brain through a different use of the Watcher.

The first phase of rebuilding involved many of the exercises I had done earlier to repair the body, and they helped. (I will teach you all of these methods in what follows here.) But there was still the problem of the lost memories. How was I to regain those?

In my usual level of consciousness, I had lost huge amounts of information. I used to teach literature, but now I couldn't even remember the names of authors and novels and poems, let alone all the other information I had amassed. I could not remember any of the research I had been doing, even though I had been an "expert" in my field, called on as an external examiner for PhD degrees and the like. I had been working on a biography of a 19th century writer but could not remember any of the information about the life of the person about whom I had hoped to write. I had even lost the memory of many of the key events in my own life.

That was in my everyday level of consciousness, the kind which depended on brain function to work. A neuropsychologist at the university confirmed, with many tests, that the area of the brain where this information was stored had been so badly damaged by the encephalitis that there was little likelihood that I would be able to reclaim any of my memories.

However, using the methods of meditation I had learned earlier, I discovered that, if I switched levels of consciousness to the level inhabited by the Watcher, I could remember. But here something else of tremendous importance dawned on me. When I was in this state I was not "remembering" in the usual sense of drawing information from the storage areas of the brain. I was actually "observing" the experiences I had in the past, in the same way as I had "observed" the disintegration of the body during the Near Death Experience in 1966. I put quotes around "observing" because it was not our usual way of observing, either. The Watcher was aware in a way quite different from that of the senses or the brain. It knew everything all at once, and space and time were not barriers to its knowing.

There was another similarity with the Death Experience. While observing, from the Watcher perspective, events in which I had taken part in the past, I could also recover the feelings and attitudes and ideas that were involved in those events. I could even pick up details of the causes of the feelings, the connections to other events and experiences in the network which held them all together. And even more important, I could resolve conflicts and trauma in that state before willing the memories into my brain for later instant access. This was not epistemological knowledge. This was a complete *gnosis*, a complete recovery of everything about the experiences, and it was achieved by entering into a particular level of awareness which I found could be taught to others.

For more than ten years I spent hours and hours, daily entering into that state, observing the experience of the past, resolving any conflicts that had been stored with them and then willing the memories into the damaged brain, almost as I had willed the network patterns back into the body so that it could live again in 1966.

As I re-entered the past, I also had to re-experience the emotions, fears, anger, worry, anxiety, love, joy and happiness of those experiences. I found myself expressing the tears, laughter, anxiety and hope of those "past times" as if I was experiencing them for the first time. It was a tremendously healing experience, as all aspects of the self were finally drawn together, even all those things that had been repressed or forgotten at an earlier age.

In this level of awareness, events no longer seemed "past," but somehow concurrent with my present experience, just on another level of awareness. I had discovered something tremendously important about how human consciousness functions. On one level we have the "physical" body and brain and senses which give us instant access to memories and experience. Without them our experience in the world would not be as intense as it is.

But on another level there is the "spiritual network" which I had experienced separating from the body in 1966. This matrix, the interconnected interplay of all aspects of our lives, is a kind of psychic double of the physical life. In it are recorded, in more subtle energy form, all that we have been and have experienced and known in life. Observing on this level is not as intense as on the "physical" level, but it is more all-inclusive. And the access to this level of awareness is made through the Watcher.

Another fascinating aspect of this period of recovery from illness involved past lives. I had done work on this earlier but now, from the perspective of the Watcher, I discovered that a "past life" was like a "past spiritual network." The body from the past had died and disintegrated, but the "network" of all of its experiences, ideas and attitudes still existed and could be accessed. I could enter into the experience of what seemed "past" lives as easily as entering a memory of my childhood, because the spiritual network was not itself past.

In addition, I discovered there was a "spiritual network" at a "higher" level, where all lives were interconnected and the "Self" which perceived on this level transcended all lives. However, this transcendent Self was the same as the Watcher, so we have within our easy reach, every day, the possibility of connecting with this transcendent Self which can see all of what we have ever been.

It is not essential that you believe in reincarnation to benefit from most of the exercises in this book. Most of them are directed toward developing, in the present, all that we can be. However, there are some experiences which only make sense if reincarnation is taken into account.

I describe this matter of what "past lives" are in more detail in *The Thomas Book* where it became a very important aspect of the writing of that book. I also explore the subject in Chapter Twelve of this book. But I will mention a few aspects of reincarnation here because it was important to my spiritual development as I recovered from encephalitis. What I discovered about human consciousness during this phase of recovery, in fact, only made sense if reincarnation of some sort is the way souls learn in this and other lives.

I think of the "spiritual network" as a "field" because the network is active like a magnetic field and any change we make in one part of the field affects other parts of the field. That is why it is so easy to make changes for the better in our lives, because we do not have to change every detail. Often, changing a prejudice will change action and attitude and relationship. Changing an idea or belief can do the same. Trying to "heal the body" may have limited effectiveness, because we just heal the hand or foot, but even small changes at fundamental levels of mind or spirit can make almost miraculous changes in our whole being.

Actually, in order to heal my brain and my memories, I had to enter into past lives, because they were intricately connected in a much larger network with my present life. On the level of the individual "Bruce," I was a "soul," but on the level where I shared life with those other manifestations we call "past-lives," I was getting in touch with my "Spirit," or what we will later call "Atman/Spirit," which is one with God, the Divine Centre of our being. At higher and higher levels we are parts of more and more inclusive patterns of relationship. At the highest levels, we human beings are all one with each other and with the Divine Centre of all our beings. At these levels, Love is the tremendously powerful force which draws us all together into a co-operative whole, a Divine Oneness.

In order to bring healing and balance into my present life, I had to enter into what appeared to be "past" lives, but which I discovered were really concurrent with the present, only on a different parallel frequency – like the physi-cists talking about parallel universes. In the same way as my present body had an intimate matrix holding its pieces together, so too there was a larger matrix holding all of the relationships, ideas and experiences of my present life together -- and on a still larger level there was a more complex matrix hold-ing all my past lives together in unity. It was possible to become aware of all these levels of consciousness, bringing them into unity, until finally all things worked as one.

I discovered that, from the perspective of the Watcher, all lives in which I had a part were of equal weight or value. Because the encephalitis had de-stroyed so much of what "Bruce MacDonald" had been, I discovered that, in order to put the present "Bruce MacDonald" life back together, I also had to integrate the other lives in which I had been involved. And it was through the perspective of the Watcher, that aspect of my consciousness which had watched and participated in the death of Bruce in 1966, that I was able to gain access to all those parallel frequencies of experience.

I think you can begin to see why I spend so much time familiarizing you with the idea of the Watcher. It is through this aspect of your consciousness that you will be able to enter into the same kinds of healing and creativity I have experienced. I have become much more than the little Bruce ego which I had been before the encephalitis, and you can learn from my experience and become much more than the limited person you may think yourself to be. I will try to give you a taste of what you can become, in spite of your apparent limitations.

In terms of Yeshua's teachings, I had been able to enter consciously into the inner Kingdom of God, the spiritual dimensions of consciousness which we all have, but which are so difficult to explain and so difficult to enter. You can now see why it would be as hard for a rich man to enter the Kingdom of God as for a camel to go through the eye of a needle (Matt 19:24). Anyone who is focused in the physical part of their nature, like money or any other element of "this present age," or anyone who is tied to the ego and its identification with what the body is worth in terms of social position or political power or the like, will find it almost impossible to find their way into the parallel "Kingdom" of our spiritual nature which transcends all our little ideas of ourselves.

I can truthfully say, with Yeshua, that my Kingdom is not of this world. I have experienced the spiritual wasteland the world can be when we try to live only in its terms. I know that I am not my body or my social position or my brain or my possessions. My Kingdom is of another world entirely. I also know that I was much closer to the Kingdom of God as a child than when I tried to "put away childish things" and ignore the promptings of the heart and spirit.

Yeshua was right. The gate to this world is narrow, indeed. It is hard to find, and those who find it are few. But for those who do find it, this Kingdom is worth all our wealth and position, and once we know of it, we would give all we have to buy the field in which we might find this pearl of great price. Once we do find it, this secret ingredient provides the best salt and yeast and flavour for the best bread of life possible. If you seek only the things of this world, that is all you will ever have. But if you seek the Kingdom of God, you will have Love and Joy and Peace in abundance, along with all the material things you need to support life.

***

The perennial flowers of the soul

I now understand that my whole life has been involved in spiritual transformation and the development of spiritual perception and awareness. It has been an extremely effective, if often painful, spiritual education. As you can see, it came in stages.

As I have already said, the process really became focused in about 1981 when Yeshua asked me in meditation if I was willing to enter a "training program." He said I could stop any time I wanted if it became too difficult. I agreed, not realizing what it would involve or how difficult it would become. But interestingly, even at the most difficult, I had a sense of being supported in what I was going through. Even following the collapse of my life after the encephalitis, at the deepest levels, I knew I would be okay.

I am assured by my Inner Guides that the program will not be as hard for others entering it, because I have been able to walk the path first and find what can make it easier for those who come later. As with all spiritual programs, the more people who enter, the easier it becomes, because we can draw on the insights of others, on the "morphogenetic field" (as Rupert Sheldrake calls it) which is established by those who have discovered the road through the wilderness of the small self.

Out of this intense education in the nature of consciousness, the present volume has arisen. Its lessons will help you, also, to become a Dweller in Two Worlds.

As I said earlier, the training program I had entered turned out to be very ancient, stretching back through Yeshua to Elijah and Moses, who I had met in the Near Death Experience in 1966, back through the schools of the prophets and even beyond. But that is not to say that there is a cause and effect, historical continuity to this program. You do not have to find documented evidence of influences from one person to the next and the next through time. That is because this program is not really in time at all.

Let me explain. What I am teaching here is part of what has been called the Perennial Philosophy. Sometimes it is called Hermetic or mystical philosophy. In many ways it is the kind of thing Socrates taught, before Aristotle turned philosophy into a matter of following a strict, logical, cause and effect sequence through time. It found a voice in poets like William Blake or in philosophers like Emanuel Swedenborg and Meister Eckhart. In the 19th century it found its voice in Helena Blavatsky and the Theosophical movement, although resistance to it was so strong at that point that its voice became muted and distorted, even in the present, although her books are well worth reading.

The reason it is called the Perennial Philosophy is that it is like flowers which come up every year, even when it seems like they have died during the season of dormancy. They pop up in the most unlikely places. Why? Because they are rooted in our deepest nature, in the soul-memory which we carry from life to life. You can learn some of this philosophy, this "Love of Wisdom," through epistemological study, but the most important parts can only be learned in your experience, in *gnosis*, in "heart knowledge" rather than "brain knowledge."

This Kingdom of God is not outside, like books or arguments or historical events. Rather, this Kingdom of the Divine One is within you, and it is by looking within that you will find it. For this reason, there are no doctrines here.

The program may be ancient but is also new for each person following it. You will find your own truth, but you will also find that, at the deepest levels, we all share the same truths. Do not try to put those truths into laws, because that is merely the ego trying to assert that it has "finally" found the truth and wants to enforce it on others. Each person must find his/her own meaning, re-creating the ancient wisdom within them. This truth will not enslave you: as Yeshua said, this truth will set you free in a most wonderful way.

However, there are values involved in this search. Love, joy, peace, kindness, gentleness, generosity, helpfulness, compassion, sharing and anything which tends to overcome divisions is helpful in the search.

As soon as hatred, violence, revenge, anger, greed, lust, domination, exclusion and the like enter into life, all spiritual progress stops until you resolve those feelings and move back to love.

If you read the two lists of values I have just given, you will sense a change in yourself just by reading the words. Use that feeling as a guide in your progress. Test your ideas and actions with those lists. If you are approximating the first list, you are in the right way. If you are moving into the qualities in the negative second list, you need to re-examine yourself and resolve some serious issues. That is the only "doctrine" in this Kingdom of God.

The program was especially difficult for me, because I was being taken from the modern way of seeing the world, into a completely different way without any external teachers or books to guide me. I had to learn everything within the inner Kingdom itself. In order to teach me what was possible, my Inner Teachers had to lead me through the most severe difficulties and let me discover the way the ancient teaching program could solve the problems. Not everyone, thankfully, has to follow my path. You can enter the program without having to fall down holes or get encephalitis, because this book (and others) presents the ancient wisdom in ways which can avoid some of the hardship.

The witness of all the great enlightened ones, including Yeshua, has been that "God is within you." If they could find this awareness of God, they say, we also can find the Divine within us. You will find your own Inner Teacher, for it will be as God said through Jeremiah,

"I will put My law in [your] minds, and write it on [your] hearts; and I will be [your] God, and [you] shall be My people. No more shall every man teach his neighbour, and every man his brother, saying, 'Know the Lord,' for [you] all shall know me, from the least of them to the greatest of them, says the Lord. For I will forgive [your] iniquity, and [your] sin I will remember no more." (Jer 31:33-34)

We are being called to a different kind of awareness. This inner awareness cannot be found by strictly rational thought, although reason and learning are very important. Ignorance breeds only more ignorance. Violence breeds only more violence.   The mind finally becomes trapped in its theories and doctrines, in its judgements and condemnations, in its fear and hatred.   More theories and more hatred will get us nowhere.   The only way out of this morass is to turn within, to find Love and Joy and Peace within and to discover that the real meaning of life is found within us.

As I look back, I realize that my search since childhood has born fruit. Was it worth it? It is worth everything. As Yeshua says, if a man discovers there is a pearl of great price in a field, he will sell everything and buy that field so that he can have the most valuable thing he can think of. It is indeed something for which one would give absolutely everything.

Perhaps even more encouraging, I have discovered through counselling those in need and through teaching others about this meditation that this spiritual awareness is open to anyone who is willing to spend time each day in the Inner Silence.

In spite of the prevailing materialism of our society, which claims that nothing spiritual is real, I know from experience that Yeshua is very real and can be contacted through the inner senses. Elijah and Moses are also real and some of what I have learned here has come from them. There is a continuing realm of spirit in which all of these great teachers function. They are part of what St. Paul called "a great cloud of witnesses" (Hebrews 12:1). These witnesses include all the people who have left the physical life and have gone into the world of spirit. Some of them were advanced enough that they could continue to help those in the flesh.

The door to that realm of spirit is within us. This is part of what Yeshua called the Kingdom of God, the realm to which we can gain access in a variety of ways. Many people have had Near Death Experiences or other spiritual experiences where they have sensed the presence of God or of Yeshua or even of their "dead" relatives.

Yeshua knew children often had access to this realm. He also knew that for people immersed in materialism it was almost impossible to explain what this Kingdom of God is, but that once you had a variety of stories pointing to it, you could begin to get a sense of what he was talking about. I have done the same thing in this chapter. I have told you a number of stories or have explained some ideas which point to this Kingdom of God and what it means. I hope you have gotten a glimpse of what this Kingdom is, because now we will enter into an active exploration of that realm where we meet God within us.

I hope that by the time you have finished reading this book and trying some of the exercises in it, you will be like the prophets of old who had such a sense of the Divine Presence within and around them that they could talk to God "as a man talks to his friend." I hope you will have become much more aware of the richness of your spiritual nature and how it impacts on your life and relationships in the world.

As you enter into yourself and discover the Divine "Kingdom of God" which is there, you will also find that the very act of being aware of the inner love, joy and peace automatically enriches the outer life we all live together on this planet, to create a society of love, joy and peace.

Chapter Five

Initiation – Getting to know the Watcher and the Self

As you practise the Prayer of Silence, you will find that a profound change in orientation takes place in your life. This will not be merely a change in ideas or in beliefs. By going beyond theory or the ideas in the mind, through the actual practise of the Prayer of Silence, you will begin to see yourself and the world differently. This is because you will begin to discover, in your own experience, that there really is another world in which you can live – a world of the Spirit.

In our everyday lives, we are usually oriented outward. We live there, act there and have relationships there. Even when we read and think, we are not actually looking at the world within -- we are only moving ideas around in the mind, as if they are objects. Thus, we argue over the "objectivity" of our ideas and our views. We want them to be as real as we think objects are.

In the Prayer of Silence, we enter another world -- the one within us. It seems at first less real than the outer one but, in time, we learn that the insights we gain there are of great value for our total life. As we persevere in our practice, this inner world begins to blossom and the experience of this inner world becomes rich and varied.

We usually think that the outer world is what makes us as we are -- that the world is the cause of what is within us. *The Prayer of Silence* demonstrates, in a very real way, that the opposite is true: we have mistaken the cause for the effect. What we are within us causes the world to be as it is. That is because the inner world is the source of all creativity from which we actually manifest our experience in the outer world – positive and negative.

So, we argue here that it does not help to change the world without first changing what is within us: in fact, it is impossible to change the world first. The world changes when we human beings change within.

The Prayer of Silence, then, is a means of focussing within, focussing on the real causes of life, so that, having found what is there, we can build on the good we see within and correct the errors we find.

The inner world is very complex and the doors to the inner country are hard to find without help and guidance. This book is a guide for finding the keys to the doors of the Self.

The Prayer of Silence is taught first as certain ideas and techniques for entering the Silence of the Self and the Silence of God. The word "Silence" is used because, when we are in the Silence, we can leave behind the noise and distraction of the outer world for a time and be aware of other dimensions of our being. Once the techniques of entering the Silence have been learned and made part of our awareness, we can then move on to build a sense of who we are and who we can become.

This book also has an important aim beyond meditation techniques. The ideas we hold in our minds and the beliefs we have about the world, have a profound effect on our lives. For that reason, this book also explores a number of important ideas which will make it easier for most readers to understand what is happening to them as they progress on the inner way. Our introductory discussion of the many aspects of the Kingdom of God in Yeshua's teachings, for instance, has given us a general picture of how the Prayer of Silence can affect the whole of life. Now we need to put the theory into practice.

Although what I call "The Prayer of Silence" is similar to meditation and draws on many meditative traditions, it is also a prayer, a conversation with God, the Divine Reality and the Presence we find within and around us as we enter the Silence. This practise of the Prayer of Silence moves us from our usual feeling of separation from the divine, to an experience of, and then an absolute certainty of our Oneness with God.

God, we will discover, is to be found within the Self -- or as Yeshua says, "The Kingdom of God is within you" (Luke 17:21). Where better than in the Kingdom to find the "King"? But finding this kingdom is not about political power, as suggested by the term "King." It is qualified by parables which say that the inner knowing is like experiencing the flavour which salt adds to food or which yeast adds to bread. It is like the pearl of great price for which we would give everything. It is like something we would clean our whole house to find.

In order to overcome the sense of separation from God which most people (even most religious people) experience, it is important to develop this interior sense of the Divine Presence. This will likely take some time, but be patient: it is entirely possible, in spite of our conditioning which often says that we cannot possible know God.

Almost all our religious traditions have tended to place the Divine outside of us, in a Heaven or Paradise or the sky or somewhere away from where the most important aspects of our lives seem to occur. So, we think we have to go to a particular place of worship to find God, or we have to listen to a particular holy person to learn of God, or we have to leave our work and relationships to find God, or we have to bow in a particular direction or sit just so, in a particular way. And often we are taught that there has to be an "intermediary" between us and God, whether this is a priest, a saint, a mullah, a rabbi, an angel or even Yeshua.

This sense of distance from God is due partly to the way we use language to describe our spiritual nature. We often think we "have a soul" which an external God somehow "made" to be "inside" us. So we think of the Divine as a controlling, creating force somehow separate and outside or above our physical life, like a potter making a pot.

When we talk of prayer, then, we often think of it as being directed to this outside deity. We think we have to direct our prayers in a particular direction so they will "get to" God, almost like tuning an aerial so that radio waves will get to the divine receiver. Often we feel we cannot approach God in the darkness of our life -- it wouldn't be right, many think, to pray in a toilet or in a barn while looking after the cattle!

But the experience of all the meditative traditions has been that God is to be found within, wherever we happen to be. Even the most squalid prison is an appropriate place to enter the Silence of God.

We can take this one step further. Not only is God always available, because the Kingdom of God is always within us, wherever we go, but we need to realize that we are actually an expression of God or a manifestation of the divine reality. The biblical writers expressed this idea by saying we are "in the image of God" (Gen 1:26).

If we are somehow an expression of God's reality, however limited we may think we are, then what Yeshua says makes sense, that the nearest place to find God is within us. But additionally, if we are an expression of the divine reality, then we cannot be as limited as we usually think we are. Somehow, we have been led to believe we have limits which we really do not have. We have been told over and over about our "sinful nature," or about our "fallen nature." But the biblical insistence that we are "in the image of God," asserts that we do not have a sinful nature – rather, error is something which is added onto our basic divine nature and error can always be corrected.

Again, part of our problem is language. Most languages are poor in their vocabulary for describing spiritual things. I found over the years that many of the available words did not adequately describe my experience in this inner Kingdom of God, because the Christian tradition has tended not to accept that God is within us and so did not develop the necessary words to convey that idea. Finally, I had to look in a number of other languages and traditions for words and concepts which would express what I was experiencing, as you have seen in our discussion of the Greek word "*gnosis*" earlier in the book.

In order to develop a way of expressing this sense of the "Inner Kingdom of God," this feeling that is developed as we continue to enter the Silence of the Self and find God there, I have found it helpful to adopt some words from Sanskrit, an ancient language of India which is rich in words describing spiritual experience.

When you say, "God," there are so many different associations which arise in the mind. Many people will not even use that word to speak of the Divine because it is so loaded with other meanings and associations with groups, doctrines, emotions, comparisons which they do not like. But I have not been able to find an alternative to that word without confining myself to other traditions. If I call the Divine by names from different religions, then I am trapped by implication into those traditions. And I wish to be free of traditions and their prejudices but still to talk of the Divine in a kind of shorthand, in a generic way, using one word.

Therefore, in order to avoid misunderstanding about what I mean when I say, "God," in the following pages, and in order to understand what we will be exploring as "the Watcher," it would be helpful if we could begin to distinguish between different aspects of our spiritual nature from the outset.

What I refer to as "God" is intimately related to what we are. But God is not a person, in the way we think of a person, with limits in time and space. We may be "in the image of God," but we are also quite different in many respects.

How can we talk about the "God within us," and at the same time distinguish other aspects of our inner nature? Since you will come across many aspects of the self, including the Watcher, in your meditative explorations, it would be helpful if I gave you a brief description of the "layers of self" you will encounter.

For instance, we often speak of "body, soul and spirit" as if we had three levels of being. However, it is more complex than that.

The next meditation exercise, the one I call your initiation, will put you in touch with the most profound aspect of your awareness – the Watcher which is an expression of what I will shortly explain is the Atman/Spirit. Other exercises will get us in touch with different aspects of our bodies and the actions of our bodies in the world.

However, we know we have emotions and memories which do not seem to be aspects of our bodies. Ideas are related to our brains, but in meditation we will find that they are also accessible from the Watcher aspect of consciousness, and these memories are "stored," not only in the brain, but in every cell of our body. After the encephalitis, when my brain was badly damaged, I discovered that memories are also stored outside of the body and brain and can only be accessed in that case from the Watcher aspect of consciousness, not from the brain at all. This aspect of the self is sometimes referred to as "mind."

When you become a little more experienced, you will be able to sense a type of body around you which is not physical. It seems to be more like a magnetic field and is referred to by some traditions as the "Astral Body." In our healing exercises it will be very important to perceive this body since it is an aspect of the network or matrix I sensed as I was dying and as I was getting the body ready for life again. It was by willing a connection between the matrix/astral body and the "physical" body that I was able to get the "old machine working again."

If we keep going in our exploration of the various "bodies" which we have, we will become aware of something we might call "soul." This is what I described earlier as the self-conscious, magnetic field which moves from life to life, adding to itself, developing itself, attracting its particular qualities to itself in each lifetime.

The Watcher aspect of the self which you will experience shortly is in some ways independent of all of these. It is tremendously powerful. It is the conscious, active, evaluative, creative and organizing aspect of our highest Self – what is usually referred to as "Spirit." The Watcher is the active principle of Spirit, and Spirit is the "Being" aspect of our Divine nature. In our meditations we aim finally to be aware of "Spirit" so we can see all of life from the perspective of Spirit.

But where is God in all this exploration of our inner being? How do we find God if we just look at ourselves?

To understand the experience of God in the Silence, we must first get a sense of what this "Spirit" is that we are aiming at. In Sanskrit, Spirit is called "Atman." Since the word "spirit" has so many other connotations, including vodka, I find it helpful to adopt the more exact word "Atman" or "Atman/Spirit" to describe the highest aspect of our spiritual nature. It is at this highest level that we are "One with God." This is because this Atman/Spirit is the way God manifests in us.

But remember the quotation from *The Gospel of Thomas* where Yeshua said, "Split a piece of wood, I am there"? He was referring to the way this Divine Atman/Spirit is present even in the simplest of things – present even in the bread and wine of a meal together, which is why Yeshua's statement in introducing the "Last Supper" is so powerful. When he says of the bread and the wine, "This is my body; this is my blood," he is making us aware of how God is present even in the simplest of things on the dinner table.

Of course, we cannot describe God's Presence directly, because it is not a thing of words but of our highest inner awareness. So we need to use metaphors, comparisons or parables to understand what we are talking about.

Visualize your total, personal experience (everything about you -- body, emotions, ideas, relationships, possessions) as rays of light shining from one light-source within you. We name this Source "Atman/Spirit." My body is not Atman. My brain is not Atman. My emotions are not Atman. The life source which surrounds and interpenetrates my cells is not Atman. When you look at any aspect of your experience, you are not looking at Atman/Spirit itself but you are looking at one of the rays shining, however dimly, from this spiritual, creative centre.

Some of the rays of light are brighter than others. Some are completely dark. Both the "good" and the "bad" are creative rays, but some of those rays have been darkened to the extent that they do not seem to reflect the Divine Source at all.

Now, take this comparison a step further. Think of everything in the universe, including all the people, each having at its centre one of these Atman/Spirit "Light Sources." All your neighbours, the animals, the trees – all have the Divine Atman Light Source at their centre. In fact, it is this Light Source which makes it possible for everything to exist. It is this light "which lights everyone coming into the world" as John's Gospel puts it.

Think of all these smaller Light Sources, including your own, as being in the image of the One Source, the Divine Light.

Then think of some of Yeshua's parables about the Kingdom of God. He says the Kingdom of God is like salt which gives flavour to our lives. It is like yeast which a woman put in a lump of dough so that the whole loaf could rise. It is like a pearl of great price which we would trade everything for if we only knew it was there. It is a well of water springing up to eternal life. It is the lamp which we should not cover with a basket. Notice how, in all of these parables, the divine centre, what I have called the Light Source within us, is described as the source of our life, of our vitality, of our value, of our purpose in life. It is the Kingdom of God within us.

All of this is summed up in the word, "Atman/Spirit." It is the Atman which is the Light Source which is an expression of the Divine Source which is the salt and yeast and pearl of our life. That is what we seek to experience, so that we can also experience our Oneness with the One Source, with God.

I would take this even one step further. In the same way that our body has a centre of consciousness which unites all the various aspects of it, so the universe, all that is, has a consciousness which unites it. This Universal Consciousness is another picture of what I call God. And we can communicate with this Universal Consciousness through our own Atman/Spirit, which is an expression in miniature of that greater Consciousness.

In communicating with God, then, we are not trying to project our words out to a great distance, because God's Presence is actually the Light Source, the centre of consciousness, which is within us. And in the same way as we are centres of consciousness, and can express our feelings and ideas in words, so too this inner Light Source is conscious and can respond to us. In that way, we actually talk to God, not as a tiny part talking to the totality of God, but as a tiny part talking to the part of God which is manifest in our own lives.

These have been attempts to describe what I mean by "God." And when I say we are "communing with God," it is this sense of the indwelling, surrounding, creative, loving Presence that we are communicating with. All of that which exists has consciousness as its centre, to the extent that some physicists say that the universe is more like a giant thought than like a thing. Everything, in its own way, is conscious, and we can communicate with a part or we can communicate with the Whole -- with God. My experience has been that God will communicate in many ways, including in words which we can understand. The communication with God can be as simple as a few words heard by a child, Samuel, in the temple night, or as simple as the "still, small voice" which Elijah heard, or which you can hear.

Of course, God is much more than we can ever hope to comprehend. We need only get a glimpse of the stars and nebulae in the universe to know that we cannot begin to feel close to the Cause of this infinite universe, much less describe or understand this aspect of God with our earth-bound brains. But God is also manifest in each of us in our Spirit, in Atman. It is not an impossible task to know this Atman, and through that knowing, to know God.

So, when we talk to God in the Prayer of Silence, we are not directing our words into infinite space or far away in a Heaven of some sort or toward some point on the earth: we are communing with God in the most essential part of our Selves. Atman and God, the Light and its Source, are One. As we become aware of that oneness, we begin to experience the greatest bliss.

Different traditions have used other metaphors to try to describe this experience of Oneness. Some say that Atman/Spirit is like a drop of water in the ocean — distinct yet one with the ocean. In accounting for my own experience in meditation, I find the metaphor of Atman/Spirit being a Ray of Light of the Divine Sun helpful because, in visualizing this metaphor, I have the sense of the Divine Sun central to my being, and then I can see my life as the shining of that light to the world. The Jewish mystical writers speak of the Atman/Spirit as being a Spark of the Divine Fire, with the whole universe as the Fire of God. John's Gospel draws on this ancient tradition when he says that the Divine Light "was the true Light which lights everyone coming into the world" (John 1:9).

St. Paul expresses it another way. He tells the Athenians, "For in him [God] we live and move and have our being; as certain of your own poets have said, for we are also his offspring" (Acts 17:28). Here Paul explains that we live and move and have our being within God. But in writing to the Corinthians he goes even farther by claiming that God is also in us: "Know you not that you are the temple of God, and that the Spirit of God dwells in you?" (I Cor. 3:16). For Paul, God is in us and we are in God.

Paul expresses this idea again to the Colossians: "God's plan is to make known his rich and glorious secret which he has for all peoples. And the secret is that Christ is in you, which means that you will share in the glory of God . . . With all possible wisdom we warn and teach them, in order to bring each one into God's presence as mature individuals in union with Christ" (Col. 1:27-28).

When Paul refers here to Christ, the "*Christos*," he is not speaking only of Yeshua, although he speaks of Yeshua as an expression of the *Christos*. The

Christos is the *Logos*, (see John 1) the essential Meaning, Light and Being of God in the universe. It is through the *Logos* that the universe comes into being. John says in his Gospel that Yeshua is the *Logos*, the Word. Paul makes a further claim. Paul says that the *Logos*, the essential being of God, is within us. We, like Yeshua, arise from *Logos* or *Christos*. We can, he claims, move toward "union with Christ," union with the *Logos*, the very essence of God.

For Paul, then, the spiritual process was one of bringing people into a *gnosis* of, an experience of union with the *Logos*, the Christ. Yeshua and Paul are not teaching a religion of correct doctrines and beliefs here. Rather, they are leading their disciples to an actual awareness of God within and around them, and that is what I wish to do through this book.

In these and other places, Paul explains in a variety of ways that we can never be separated from God because we are of the very nature of God. What we are here calling the Atman/Spirit as the expression of God in us, Paul calls the "*Christos*," the indwelling presence and being of God. Much of Paul's teaching involves the development and growth of this indwelling *Christos* (Atman) to bring us to spiritual maturity.

But again, because the word "Christ" has so many varied meanings in so many churches, I will still use the term "Atman/Spirit" to express this idea of the *Christos/Logos*. There is an important distinction in philosophy in the changed emphasis.

Most Christian churches (and other religions) teach that it is merely by "believing in Jesus" or "believing in the power of the blood" or "believing in the correct doctrine," or believing in something similar to these, that we are "saved." What we believe certainly makes a difference in how we live our lives, but beliefs in themselves do not somehow "save" us from ourselves.

Paul's message, and the message of the Prayer of Silence, is that we actually "become Christ." We become one with God as we seek daily, throughout our lives, to allow the deeper Love, Joy and Peace of God, the Atman/Spirit which is at the centre of our being, to shine like a Divine Sun into our lives and into the world around us.

All these metaphors assert that it is from the very life of God that we spring. So it is not so difficult for us to find God as "Our Father," (to use another metaphor) as Yeshua instructs. "Our Father" is closer to us than the skin on our fingers, since we are, in our innermost being, God. Or as Yeshua says, "Know you not that you are gods" (John 10:35).

You can see why it is important to get an exact sense of what I mean when I say, "God," since there are many other understandings of what or who God is and what our relationship to the Divine is like. In entering the Silence, in carrying on this inner communication, we can "talk to God," not as talking to ourselves and not as talking to some being separated from us in a different realm, but as talking to the very Source from which we have come and to which we return and which we are.

However, in the beginning we will start more simply than this. We will deal with our bodies and feelings and ideas and relationships. They are an expression of what we have done with the inner Light of Atman as it shone through our being. Sometimes we will find God in our lives, but often we will find that we have darkened the Light until it is unrecognizable as the Ray of God's Light. So we have to continue on the road back to the Light.

***

Meeting the Watcher for the first time

In most of the chapters, I suggest a variety of exercises which will gradually bring you to a realization of your spiritual nature. These exercises are designed to gently awaken a particular awareness of your inner being. It is important that you practise them and not just read about them. Reading will only give you *episteme*: practise will give you *gnosis*. Of course, you may want to read the whole book to get an overview of the ideas, but then make sure you come back and practice the exercises. This book is not just about information.

You may also think that since you have used other meditative techniques, you can skip these. I have taught the techniques included here to people who have spent many years using other methods and they have found that what is presented here has added a great deal to their practise. These exercises are actually designed to open certain spiritual abilities and senses gradually and it helps if you do them in the order suggested here. They are not just haphazard exercises.

You should especially do the exercise which introduces you to the Watcher. The rest of the book will be meaningless without the actual experience of entering into that central consciousness, because the rest of the exercises depend on it. Even if you only succeed a little bit in becoming aware of the

Watcher, that will be a help. Most people will find it quite easy to enter into that level of awareness.

You have been gradually becoming aware of the way you spend your day and night by doing the exercise designed to bring that into focus. However, at the same time you have been learning about the day, you have also been developing an ability to relax and to focus your attention on memories, feelings, ideas and events. It may look like you have been looking outward but you have actually been looking within yourself. Some of you may even have found things which needed changing and so your lives have changed through this process of inner reflection.

You have also been able to stop for a moment in your day and have learned to project your awareness outward into the natural landscape or into a room full of people. You have thus learned another way of being aware of the world around you and you may have begun to perceive things about the world which you could not have perceived without stopping in that way to sharpen the focus of your awareness and to expand it beyond yourself.

Now I would like to introduce you to the Watcher aspect of your consciousness, the same aspect I encountered in the Near Death Experience. Just to remind you, this is the "centre of consciousness" from which I observed all that was happening to my body and memories and feelings as the physical part of the life which had been Bruce came to an end. It was also the "centre of consciousness" from which I was able to put the memories and life force back into the body to get "the old machine" to work again. It is both an observer of events in our total being as well as the source of tremendous creative power, as you will find in exercises later in the book.

The Watcher is actually intimately related to the exercises you have already been doing and they will make it easier for you to perceive this centre of awareness within you. One of the great philosophers of the Hindu tradition, Shankara, who taught what is known as "Advaita" (non-dualism), was very aware of this Watcher aspect of the self. He called it Atman, as we have been doing. Someone asked him one day where this Atman was to be found and he said, "You use it all the time, but are not aware of it." Most people do not become aware of this aspect of consciousness (often because their teachers are not aware of it), until they have spent many years in meditation. Many other traditions are obviously not even aware that there is anything like the Watcher to discover, even though it is the most used aspect of our being.

It may even seem that it is a bit too advanced to teach this most subtle of states of awareness this early in our practice. Most meditative systems start with something simple, like concentrating on the breathing or repeating a "mantra." Only after much repetition is the person made aware of the Watcher/Atman, if at all. We start differently here because I want you to become aware of the most important "sense" in meditation from the start. We can build from there. Interestingly, you will find getting acquainted with the Watcher both surprisingly simple and extremely complex.

I have mentioned that death and meditation are similar in many ways since, in both, we are taken out of our normal world into another realm of consciousness. It is interesting that, in the initiation rituals of the ancient Mystery Religions, of the Masonic Lodge, of many tribal societies as well as in the baptism rituals of John the Baptiser (the Jewish reformer) and in baptism in Christianity, the experience of initiation is always compared to "death."

Initiation is a way of dying to the old reality and moving into a new. This is almost always seen as a symbolic act in formal religious practice.

However, it is not always symbolic. In many aboriginal cultures, the shaman, who is the healer, priest and counsellor of the tribe, goes through a journey to the world of the spirits before he/she is able to carry on the role of intermediary between the worlds of ordinary life and the world of the spirits. Many people think the Great Pyramid was actually an initiation hall and that the sarcophagus was the "tomb" in which the initiate lay in order to experience the movement into the other world and become a "dweller in two worlds." The initiates in these cases actually had the equivalent of a Near Death Experience which was not symbolic but a literal journey into the "other world."

The initiation through which I will take you is not symbolic. It is a literal change of consciousness in which you can experience some of the qualities of the awareness which follows what we erroneously think of as "death" or termination. No one ever dies. Life is not terminated. We just change our level of consciousness when the body stops functioning -- and we can achieve that shift of consciousness in life as well as in death.

***

Meditation Exercise: Your initiation into the Watcher

This exercise will take you into the realms beyond death, where you discover that you are a spiritual being expressing aspects of your nature in a physical body. I do not want you to think of this experience as in any way symbolic. In this exercise, you will experience directly an aspect of your spiritual nature which survives your physical death. You will enter into a Kingdom not of this world. And when, many years from now, the time comes for you to leave this physical body to enter fully into the Divine Presence, you will be in familiar territory because you will have experienced much of the process already. This experience is what the symbolic initiations of baptism and ritual cleansing are actually dramatizing.

Read over the following instructions a number of times so they are familiar. Then put the book aside and enter the Silence.

In order to do this exercise, you will need a quiet place where you can sit undisturbed for some time, first for the actual initiation, and then for a time of reflection and exploration. When you have found such a place, sit in a comfortable position.

As with all the exercises in this book, start with a brief, informal talk with the Divine Source of your being which we call "God." Address your words or thoughts to this Centre of your being, not to a distant deity. Ask for guidance and support. Ask that God fill and surround you with the Divine Light and Presence.

Visualize the Light or Divine Energy around and within you. If you have any fears or anxieties, share those with God.

Then enter into the first part of the meditation which is the progressive relaxation you have already done many times. However, because this is such an important part of this exercise, I will repeat it here in detail. Read it several times so that you know the whole process and can practice it without interrupting the flow of the whole initiation.

If you are in a group, one member of the group might be the leader who leads everyone else through the exercises. And since this "initiation" can also be practiced as a continuing exercise, choose another leader the second and third time so everyone has the experience of leading and of concentrating on doing the exercise. Even if you are doing this alone, it is good to come back to this exercise many times, so that you become fully aware of the Watcher and can enter that state of consciousness easily in the future.

While you are doing the exercise, be aware of your reactions and feelings in a detached way. Try to remember what you have perceived, positive and negative. As I have emphasized before, but must especially emphasize here, your aim is not to "space out" or go into a trance, but to develop a relaxed awareness. If you go into a trance with this exercise you will have to return and do it again in order to benefit from the Watcher awareness.

Close your eyes and consciously relax your whole body for a few seconds, moving your awareness around to sense any places which especially need relaxing. Shift your body around until you feel comfortable and balanced without strain. Expect this exercise to take quite a bit longer than normal. Make sure you are comfortable and that you will not be disturbed while you are doing it. If you think you might be disturbed, choose another opportunity to do the exercise when you have sufficient time to complete it in one sitting.

Breathe deeply and pay attention to your breathing, counting each breath from one to four as you breathe in and out.

Do that for a little while until you feel quite relaxed, with the refreshing energy from your breath moving freely through your body.

Pray silently a prayer to the effect of, "God, I seek in entering this Silence to become aware of your Presence, which Yeshua assures us is always with us, and also to become aware of the centre of perception which is known as the Watcher. I ask for the presence of the Christ and your protective Light during this time in the Silence. I pray that all negative energies or forces be excluded from my time in the Silence."

You are asking for inner guidance and making it clear to yourself and to those who can help you that it is Christ's Way, the Way of the *Logos*, of the Light, of Love that you want to follow. That is important, because there are other directions and other guides on the Inner Way with which you may not be familiar. There are also negative forces which would like very much to pervert your spiritual practice and turn it to harm. You need God's Presence to guide and protect you at all times.

If you really do not know if you believe in God, even at this point, you should be honest and say something to the effect, "I really don't know if you are there at all, God, or if I am just talking to myself again. Maybe you are around, and maybe I will perceive you one of these days. Just in case you are there, please help me to find you. And during my time in the Silence I ask that your Presence be the only Presence which has any influence on me."

Above all, be honest in what you say. As we have said before, you must base this whole process on as much honesty as possible.

Now concentrate on relaxing your body in a progressive way.

Relax your face first by being aware of all the muscles in your face and by willing that they all relax.

Move your attention to the top of your head and will the muscles to relax. (pause between each step)

Relax the back of your head. (pause)

Move your attention to the sides of your head, sense your ears in the middle and will that the muscles relax. (pause and continue to pause after each step)

Let that relaxation and attention radiate into the centre of your head, until it reaches a point in the centre of your head, and then allow the relaxation to generalize into your whole face and head.

Now let the relaxation and your attention move down into your neck and flow into your shoulders like a warm liquid.

Let the relaxation and attention move into your upper arms:

-- into your lower arms to the wrists:

-- into your hands and fingers and thumbs.

Move your attention and the relaxation back to your shoulders.

Move your attention and relaxation to your upper back,

-- to your chest,

-- to your lower back,

-- to your belly.

Let the relaxation and attention flow to the base of your spine and into the area of the hips.

Let it flow into your legs, down to the knees. Feel the relaxation in the knees.

Will that the relaxation and attention move to the lower part of your legs down to the ankles.

Let it flow into your feet and toes.

Now feel any remaining tension flow out of your body, from the top of your head, through your neck, your arms and hands, your shoulders and chest, your belly and hips, down through your legs and feet and into the earth below you. (Imagine the tension and tiredness flowing from you like a warm liquid being absorbed and transmuted by the earth.)

Relax you whole body, being aware of your whole body. Do not fall asleep. You want to remain relaxed and attentive.

Now, feel the breathing coming in and going out again, in and out of your relaxed body. Concentrate on the breathing for a short while.

Then, in your imagination, surround yourself with a cocoon of light or a field of energy.

Be aware of the energy around you. Be aware of your breathing going in and out slowly. Be aware of your body within the light/energy around you, with the breath as a movement between your body and the light/energy field which surrounds you.

Now it is time to be aware of your own consciousness. Notice how you can be aware of the body. Then notice how you can move your awareness outside the body, in the space around the body. Then notice how the awareness can be directed to the breath which is flowing through the nose and lungs and also in the air which surrounds you. Notice how you are aware of the interconnectedness of all that is in and around the body.

Without disturbing the peaceful awareness of this interaction, become aware of the place from which you are viewing your body. Be aware of your left foot and then be aware of the place from which you sense this foot. Move your awareness to your right hand and then be aware of the place from which you are viewing the hand. When you are aware of the breath, from what position, in relation to the body, do you view the breath?

Ask yourself where you are "looking from" when you focus your attention. You will discover that you are not looking from your finger itself when you are focusing on your finger. Your attention comes from some other area of your body or even from outside your body. Many people find the source of their attention is behind them or to one side. It may come from the heart area, from behind the neck or from the head, but if you direct your attention toward the heart or the head you will discover a separation between the source of your "seeing" and the part of the body you are aware of.

Spend some time now focusing on one part of the body, then on the source of your seeing. Then move to another part of the body and again focus on the source of your seeing. The more you do this, the more you will get a sense of where the source of your seeing is.

Also, as you move your awareness around and as you develop a growing sense of where your attention is centred, be aware that this centre of consciousness is the Watcher I have been telling you about.

As you do this, you may also begin to get some different sensations. You may get tingling or numbness in your body. You may have a sense of floating. At times it might be as if you "shift" into another frequency of awareness.

It will not likely happen at this point, but at some time in your practise you may get the feeling that you are expanding larger and larger until you fill the whole room or the whole world with your awareness. This is called the "large body" awareness, in which you realize that the "Source" from which you are seeing, the Watcher, is not limited to the body. Do not be alarmed with any of these experiences. Just observe them and enjoy them. They are aspects of the experience of the Watcher. You will return to your body when you are ready.

As you do this exercise, you will gradually become aware that you are not your brain and that your awareness does not come from your brain. And, strange as it may seem at this point, the Source of your awareness, the Watcher, is actually the Atman/Spirit we have been talking about. You will discover that it is beyond emotion or ideas or beliefs or fears. In future exercises you will be able to look on any of your fears or beliefs or ideas from the perspective of the Watcher and you will be able to examine them without fear or judgement. You will be able to heal from this perspective, because it is the source of your creativity. If you are an artist or writer you will be able to create your art from this Source more effectively than if you try to do it from the limited perspective of the emotions or intellect.

In order to write this book I have often entered into the Watcher and have allowed the ideas to form within the Watcher field of awareness before writing them down, because I actually had to "see" the condition or the effect I was trying to describe before I could find the appropriate words to express it.

As you do this, you might remember my experience in the Near Death Experience. When I was getting ready to leave the body when it was dying, and again, when I was rebuilding the connection between Watcher and body in order to prepare it for re-entry, my awareness was not just "looking" as if from outside. It was as if the awareness of the Watcher was inside and around the body at the same time. Try to get the sense of being "inside and around" your right foot for a while. Then try the same thing with your left hand. Move your awareness around to many parts of your body in the same, inclusive way.

Another experiment to introduce at some time is to expand the Watcher awareness to your whole body and then shrink it to a hand and then expand it to surround your whole body then shrink it to a foot, then expand it to fill the whole room in which you sit then shrink it to your face. Practice this kind of plasticity of the Watcher. You have already been doing this in the exercise where you project your awareness into the world around you, except now you know what you were doing then.

In the last chapter, I will explore the experience you may have at some point in which you are one with all that is. You can do this because the Atman/ Spirit which manifests as the Watcher is one with God – or as Yeshua says, "I and My Father are one." In certain states of awareness you can be aware of how the divine centre in you is one with the divine centre in all things. It is a wonderful experience which comes as a gift once or twice in your lifetime.

During the Near Death Experience, the Watcher was just above my left shoulder, looking down at the body. For many years after that I "saw" everything in my life from just above my left shoulder. As my awareness changed, the position of the Watcher changed to reflect my growing spiritual consciousness.

Now I have learned that I can move the Watcher consciousness around, sometimes to great distances or into the past in order to do healing of others or to explore aspects of other lives.

It is from this simple beginning that you will start to become aware of the tremendous mobility and power of your spiritual consciousness.

Spend some time exploring this Watcher consciousness through the simple act of moving your awareness to different parts of the body. Sense the feeling of freedom which you have as you move at will from toe to head to finger.

You have entered into the realms beyond our ordinary physical life and its concerns. You will never again be absolutely bound by any of the worries or anxieties of the physical life, because you know that you are no longer just physical. You are a spiritual being capable of moving, in however limited a fashion now, beyond the usual awareness of the limiting senses of the body. You have entered into the realms experienced in death without dying.

Most important, you are now a Dweller in Two Worlds and can never again be fooled into thinking of yourself as just a physical body or its possessions or its position in society. This is perhaps the easiest way of freeing yourself from the limits of the personal ego.

Spend some time experiencing the wonder of this awareness, moving your awareness, experiencing the freedom of it and the new perception of it. It would be good for you to make a regular practise in the morning and evening of coming into the Silence and exploring the Watcher aspect of yourself. The more you do this, the greater discoveries you will make about the abilities of the Watcher. This is the foundation of all the other exercises in this Prayer of Silence, so practise it often and learn it well. There is no need to hurry, and this is a very productive time for the recuperation of your body and soul, so accept it and enjoy it.

When you feel you have been in the Silence for long enough and you are ready to come to full, alert consciousness again, say a word of thanks for all your have experienced, then focus your awareness back into your body, allow your mind to sweep through your body from toes to head, wiggle your fingers and toes and open your eyes.

But do not immediately get up and go about your business. Sit with your eyes open looking at the world around you. Feel the contrast of the experience you have had in the inner being and the perception you now have through the senses. See if you can see the world through the eyes of the Watcher. Project your awareness into different aspects of the apparently physical world around you. Do not rush. Observe gently and peacefully.

Only when you have finished your observations should you get up and go about your business, but carry the peacefulness and observation with you. You have changed in this short time. Be aware of the change.

You must do the exercise and not just read about it if you would reap its benefits and awareness. Everything which follows in this book depends on your having entered into the Watcher.

***

It is helpful to continue your review of the day exercise as before, but now you can add the Watcher exercise to it twice a day, morning and evening.

With practice in this Watcher exercise, you will find you can do it more and more effortlessly, until you can close your eyes and in a matter of a couple of minutes you will be completely relaxed and have a sense of a surrounding well-being and an alert awareness of what you focus your attention on. You will also develop an awareness of what the Watcher is capable of doing, how it can move, what it can perceive. All of this will make it possible to enter more effectively into the transformation exercises which follow in this book.

You will also begin to notice, as you learn to relax and perceive the Watcher aspect of the Self, that the outer world will change. You won't try so hard to define yourself by what you own or how you appear in other people's eyes and you won't worry so much whether you are doing everything according to what you think are the expectations of others. You will begin to become more self-assured in a quiet way. And you will not have to judge others so much, when you do not judge yourself so harshly. Life will become a lot easier as you give less power to the ego, the inner slave driver we all have to struggle with.

Remember to concentrate on your body at this stage. It is through your ability to be aware of the body, from the perspective of the Watcher, that you will be able to move into other areas of awareness. The body reflects, in physical form, what we need to learn spiritually, so it is essential to get to know the body and its symbolism and its ways of communicating if you wish to grow spiritually.

We do not seek to escape the body or to deny the body by entering the Watcher consciousness -- that would be self-defeating. We are, after all, in the flesh, and it is in this arena we have to learn about ourselves.

One of the sayings which can be very helpful and which emphasizes that the divine patterns of cause and effect in the universe have brought us where we are now is:

"We are where we need to be to learn what we need to learn!"

This is essentially a statement of faith in the appropriateness of the relationship between our inner being and our outer life, between the needs of our spiritual state and the possibilities of our spiritual evolution. If you meditate on "where you are" in life and what you are experiencing right now, you will learn a great deal about yourself.

Anything that helps you along the way to developing your awareness of your body and to overcoming the problems of the body, is appropriate, so jog or swim or play tennis or walk or exercise in some way to strengthen the body and to help you become more aware of how your body is a vital part of your total being. Eat a balanced diet. Look after any medical problems when they arise. Learn from your body.

You have now had a Near Death Experience without going through the experience of death! And you can repeat this experience whenever you want. In fact, the more you practice it, the better. Interestingly, you will gradually lose your fear of death as you do this, and when your time does come to die, you will know immediately what to do because you already know this area of your being and you will know that death is merely a shift of consciousness, the kind you have been doing regularly for years!

A friend of mine was in a meditation class I taught quite a few years ago. I had taught him this simple exercise and he was fascinated with this aspect of his consciousness, especially since he was partially blind and this gave him perceptions which he could not have otherwise. He was able to expand the Watcher aspect of his consciousness to perceive things around him, even when his eyes could not see them. When he died, his wife and daughter were by his side in the hospital. His wife told me that at one point he said, "Let go of my hand. It is time." Then, staring straight ahead of him, with a most glorious smile, he repeated, "It's time," and he left them in great happiness because he was already familiar with this spiritual world from his regular meditation.

You will want to do this exercise over and over again in the next few days and weeks, until you are thoroughly familiar with the Watcher aspect of yourself. It will enrich the rest of your life because you can come to this state of awareness whenever you need to.

Although I call this aspect of consciousness, "the Watcher," you will discover, as you go through the ideas and exercises in this book, that this centre of consciousness does not just watch. It can be creative, active and very mobile. It is through this consciousness that I was able to heal my body and put my brain back together. Through this consciousness you will be able to heal emotional trauma and broken relationships. Through it you will be able to create art or new perceptions.

Perhaps most fulfilling, you will also be able to start communicating with God honestly in the innermost parts of your being, beyond the delusions of the senses and the ego. It is not your brain or your body which communicates with God in this meditation -- it is the Watcher, this spiritual awareness centre, this active aspect of Atman/Spirit which communicates with the still small voice of the Divine. As you practise, this ability will grow in you as *Gnosis*, not just as theoretical knowledge.

You may want to put the book away for a few days as you practise being aware of the Watcher aspect of yourself. Experiment with moving your awareness. Try expanding your awareness by pushing the Watcher consciousness out farther and farther from your body. Try radiating light and love from yourself using the will and intention of this Watcher. Try exploring relationships. See how much you can achieve on your own before going on to the next exercise.

***

Now that you are aware of the Watcher, you will also become aware in the days and years ahead, how the Kingdom of God is within you, in the very heart of your ideas, feelings and actions. As you become aware of the negative within you, and begin to change it from the heart, you will be able to turn your darkness into light and fulfil what Yeshua says -- "You are the light of the world. . . Nor do they light a lamp and put it under a basket, but on a lamp stand, and it gives light to all who are in the house" (Matt 13:14-15). You may even begin to sense some of the intense Divine Love and Joy and Peace which have been hidden in unawareness for a long time, and which you can radiate to others.

After your initiation into the Watcher consciousness, the path we follow in the Prayer of Silence becomes clearer, because we can advance more quickly and know more fully what we are doing.

It is important now to tell God of your desire to learn. The Divine within us, the Atman/Spirit which expresses itself in the Watcher, always wants to move toward union with God. Once we express the desire to learn, we automatically activate the divine help within us which wants to move back to a sense of Oneness. We begin to awaken our own divine nature. You will awaken the inner Teacher, now that you know who you really are.

Those spiritual beings who would like to help us cannot do so unless we ask. It is forbidden for them to impose their will on us or to do our spiritual work for us. We must express our desire for enlightenment before they can help. But once we have expressed the desire, they will make their presence known in many subtle ways in our lives and in our meditations.

And finally, we will move toward the union between Atman/Spirit and our Divine Source (I discuss this union at length in the last chapter of this book). It is in experiencing this Oneness that we will find the true Love, Joy, Peace and Wisdom which come from God. God is always within us and around us and among us, so we do not have to go far to find what we seek.

Chapter Six

Practicing the Presence of God

"But my chief good is to be near you, O God,
I have chosen you, Lord God, to be my refuge."
(Ps. 73:28, RSV)

"And I will ask the Father, and he will give you another
Comforter, that he may abide with you forever;
Even the Spirit of truth; whom the world cannot receive,
because it does not see him, nor know him: but you know him;
for he dwells with you, and shall be in you."
(John 14:16-17, RSV)

You are now ready to begin "Practising the Presence of God," something that can be one of the most profound exercises in the whole, lifelong experience of the Interior Silence. You may not think that you can actually experience God's Presence with you, but it is entirely possible. And when you achieve this, you will not trade it for anything.

It may take many years of persistent effort to clear away the debris of our ego ideas of ourselves and of God before we can fully move into this area of awareness, but even in the beginning we can have success in this meditation. It is a very important area of our spiritual development, because it is here that even the simplest of people or children can participate. This is not an intellectual exercise and can be done without any education or sophisticated learning. In fact, Yeshua says, unless you become "as a little child you cannot enter the Kingdom of God" (Luke 18:17). Part of the meaning of this comment lies in the fact that children do not have all the obstacles adults have in accepting God's Presence.

This is a short chapter but one to which you should pay particular attention in developing the inner awareness.

***

Meditation Exercise: Practicing the Presence of God by paying attention to your breathing

Whenever you enter the Inner Silence, relax deeply, be aware of the body, be aware of the breath, surround yourself with the light of God and ask God for help and guidance. Nothing fancy is needed, just, "God, I'm going to be doing the breathing exercise. Please guide me into being aware of your Presence and what that can mean for me. Thanks." Again, I emphasize, stay away from a feeling that you have to be formal or that you have to use long words or theological language in your conversations with God: that only creates a distance between you and God.

Now that you know about the Watcher, you can also move your awareness to that spiritual centre within you and sense all that happens in the Silence from there. That way you are not led astray by any of your ego wants or needs.

Part of experiencing the Presence of God is related to how you address God. I am going to get you to start calling God "Abba" for this exercise. (You may want to carry that over into the rest of your life from now on, but that is not essential.) Yeshua addressed God as "Abba," "Daddy," partly, I understand, because that is how he knew God as a child, and he carried that intimate relationship over into adulthood. However, when you call God "Abba" you are not just using a substitute for "Daddy." In meditation "Abba" has a number of mystical qualities.

When you address God as "Abba" in meditation you will begin to experience a gentle, inner intimacy and absolute trust. More than friend or parent could ever be, Abba is the most personal inner presence you can experience. In this you will begin to get a sense of the sort of relationship you are working toward.

Enter into the Silence and into the Watcher as in the other exercises with which you are already familiar. Begin to breathe, except this time do not breathe unconsciously -- be aware of your breathing.

Breathe in. Feel the breath flow into your lungs, down as deep as possible without straining.

Be aware of the breath in your lungs.

Hold your breath there for a short time, for as long as is comfortable without straining, and then breath out slowly, feeling the air flow out of your body. Relax as you breathe and feel the breath flow.

Then breathe in again -- and out again, each time feeling the life energy of the air coming in and the tension and tiredness of the body flowing out with the breath.

Now become aware of perceiving the air from the perspective of the Watcher. Observe the air and the body and the interaction of the two. Sense how the air surrounds the body and how it enters into and flows out of the body. Become aware of this interaction for a while.

Once you have watched the breath and the body from the perspective of the Watcher for a little while, switch your attention and imagine that the air around you is the active agent and the air is breathing you. Feel the air as something which surrounds you and which seems to have a gentle will of its own, providing you with life and energy. Allow the air to breathe you.

Concentrate on your breathing for the time of your meditation, gradually letting yourself become aware of the air you breathe in and out as well as the air which surrounds you.

You will likely find that ideas and pictures intrude in your mind. Do not try to suppress them but say to yourself, "Ah, another idea." Then label it in your mind as a "Wandering Thought" and let it go. Then bring your mind back to your breathing. If you are like most people, you will have to bring yourself back to the breathing quite often, because the mind tends to wander. Don't worry about it. Just label the thoughts, "Wandering Thoughts," and let them wander away and bring your attention back to the body and the breath.

Because you now know how to enter the Watcher consciousness, you will likely find it is easier to meditate without wandering thoughts. The Watcher makes it much easier to maintain focus and balance.

When you have done that for ten or twenty minutes, thank God for whatever you have sensed or felt in this time of Silence, then, before you get up and start moving around again, just wiggle your fingers and toes a bit, move your arms and legs gently, stretch your whole body, and then open your eyes.

Do not shock your system by jumping up suddenly from your time in the Silence. You will discover that your consciousness and your identity is not the same as your body, although you experience through the body. When you enter the Silence, you actually achieve a slight separation between that part of your consciousness with which you perceive in the Silence (the Watcher) and the kind of awareness you have in the body. You are a little bit out of sync with the physical body so that you can perceive the energy body -- there is a difference. The more often you enter into the Silence in this way, the stronger this "energy body" becomes, by the way, and the easier it is to enter into the awareness which is built up with that energy body.

As you do this meditation, you may find that part way through the meditation it feels like you can actually sense a shift of consciousness. This shift often takes the form of a feeling of greater clarity, a sense of inner light or joy, or even a sensation of a slight "falling" into another state. This new state of consciousness is called "Samadhi" in India or "Satori" in Zen Buddhism. It is a pleasant and very productive time, so stay with it as long as you can without effort. Be thankful for that experience when you come back to ordinary consciousness.

Another experience you may have is one where your spiritual energy body seems to grow bigger than you. It can actually become very large and you seem to sense the world from a (literally) heightened perspective. Again, this is quite normal, so enjoy it and stay with it as long as you want. However, do not think that you must have these experiences. Allow them to come with gratitude and let them go with gratitude.

You may wonder why this emphasis on the breath. Why do I tell you that we will be doing an exercise which will help you become aware of the Presence of God, when all we do is sit and breathe and concentrate on the air going in and out of our lungs.

As you become more at ease with this exercise, you will be able to add another element to it which will make you gradually aware of the reason for concentrating on the breath.

In the Bible we read in Genesis that "God breathed into them the breath of Life" (Genesis 2:7). When Yeshua died, the writer says that he "Gave up the Ghost," but in the Greek text that reads, "He gave up the *pneuma* (air)" (Mat 27:50). (It is from that same source that we have *pneuma*tic tires on our cars and bicycles.)

We know from the teachings of many religions, including Judaism and Christianity, that the breath is important, both in the ordinary, everyday breathing, but also in a mystical, spiritual way.

The ancient Greeks called breath "*pneuma*," and they also called God's Spirit "*Pneuma*." The Romans breathed "*spiritus*," air, but for them God was "*Spiritus Sancti*," the Holy Spirit or Holy Air. In Hebrew the air is "*rua*," and the enfolding, maternal Spirit of God is also "*Rua*." In the Sanskrit language the life, "*jiva*," which comes from God, is in the air we breathe and is called "*prana*." However, *prana* is itself a spiritual power.

All the ancients who were familiar with the simple breathing exercise of meditation, including the spiritual ancestors of Judaism and Christianity, were also aware that this was the most direct way to be aware of the Divine Energy, the Holy Spirit. Life comes with the breath and departs with the breath, and Life comes from God.

With that in mind, let's do another exercise, which is an expansion of the one above.

***

Meditation Exercise: Sensing the Presence

Again, exactly as above, close your eyes, enter the Silence by the process of relaxing and becoming aware of your body. Become aware of seeing from the Watcher perspective by moving your awareness to different parts of the body. Ask for guidance, but this time call God "Abba" in your prayer. Be aware of the sound of that word and any feelings which go along with it. Then concentrate on your breathing from the perspective of the Watcher, in the same way you did in the above exercise.

Now, in order to add another, vital element to your meditation, you can do the simple breathing exercise, but at the same time concentrate on the sense that God is all around you, literally, and that you can feel God's Presence just as easily as you can feel the air.

As you breathe in and out, have the sense that within that air, the *spiritus*, the *pneuma*, the *rua*, the *prana*, is something more than air, something alive in a way you had not really suspected before.

God is not air, but in the sensing of the air outside and inside, you begin to become aware of another kind of Presence which is there with you.

Do not try to force anything here. You are developing a very fine sensing apparatus in your being, one that is not really part of your nerves, but is part of another system of perception related to the Watcher, one of which you will become aware of as you proceed. But you must do it gently, never frowning or concentrating with the will or the thinking mind. It actually helps if you can keep a small smile on your face while you do this, because that physical act awakens a memory of happiness which helps to perceive the Divine Presence which is Love and Joy and Peace.

Even the Watcher does not sense this Presence, although developing the Watcher helps in the process. When you sense this Presence, it is as if your whole being, including the Watcher and the Presence around you, comes together in one, total awareness. You can use your Watcher consciousness to expand your awareness into the surrounding Presence. You can "intend" your whole being to expand and enter into the Presence which is around and within you, as you did with the landscape in an earlier exercise.

As you do this, repeat "Abba" gently, being aware of talking to the "Father" of which Yeshua spoke. Say, "Abba," wait for a few breaths, say, "Abba," again and listen to the inner voice.

You may even find the experience so moving at times it will bring you to tears of happiness or to a sense of deep joy or love.

These words may not mean much intellectually or logically as you read them but, when you do the exercise, you will know what they are about. They are related to the quotation which opens this chapter. Yeshua says about the Holy Spirit, the Holy Wind, "And I will ask the Father, and he will give you another Comforter, that he may abide with you forever; even the Spirit of truth; whom the world cannot receive, because it does not see him, nor know him: but you know him; for he dwells with you, and shall be in you" (John 14:16-17).

This Holy Spirit, Holy Air, is around and within you all the time. The worldly senses do not see him or know him, but you know him now, for he dwells with you and is in you.

After the encephalitis in 1991, I was able to actually see this Presence in the form of millions and millions of small sparks of light in everything around me, almost as if the world was covered with gauze made of light. That experience kept me centred and helped me to deal with the profound loss of other functions in my life. You may sense the Presence as I do now, as an enfolding feeling almost of warmth, but with a sense of Personhood. Address this Presence as "Abba." You will gradually develop a sense of response, of love and of peace.

You may sense, rightly, that in these descriptions I am trying to give voice to what cannot be described, but only pointed to in a variety of ways. Perhaps some of the clues I give you will help you to get a sense of what is possible as you Practice the Presence.

It may take quite some time to get the sense of the Presence around you, but you are moving toward becoming what Yeshua spoke of as a person "Born of the Spirit." "Spirit" here is air in the ordinary meaning of the term, but is also Spirit in the Divine sense of "the Spirit moving upon the Waters" in Genesis. The Spirit of God breathes life into you; the Spirit of God moves around you; those born of the Spirit are like the wind and go where God's intent takes them.

God is not far away in a distant Heaven: God is within you and you are within God in a very real sense, just as you breathe the air and the air breathes you.

Don't think with the brain about God being around you. Just be aware of your breathing and the Presence around and in you. It helps greatly if you keep from thinking words when you are doing this and, if they appear, just label them "Wandering Thoughts," let them go, and return to developing your subtle awareness of the Spirit around and in you.

Do not try to interpret this sense with the mind. The mind likes to categorize and dismiss things, and it may try to tell you, "Oh, this thing you feel is just air, or just oxygen, or just some kind of magnetic field. There is really nothing to it."

When your mind does that, just treat that as if it is a Wandering Thought and let it go, bringing your attention back to the breathing and the Presence. This action is not to try to keep you from thinking or questioning but rather, to encourage you to experience what is actually there before you put mental barriers in the way.

Again, I emphasize that for most people this "Practise of the Presence" will likely take a lot of practise, but as you continue with it through the years, you will become more and more aware of God's Presence within and around you.

However, you have been preparing for this in your other meditation exercises and you may find that, after all the meditation using the Watcher as a focus, the experience of the Presence of God comes to you easily, naturally, like an extension of the Watcher itself, that centre of the Divine within you. It can be a tremendously profound experience and, in times of trial, an essential part of your practise of the Prayer of Silence and of the helping Presence of God.

This is the Breath of God within you, the Life you share with God and from which your life has arisen. It is also the basis of what the mystics call the "Unitive Vision," the Mystic Oneness, the profound sense that All is actually One in God.

***

Meditation Exercise: Advanced Presence

An advanced form of this meditation, which you can try at some point, is to gradually allow the border between you and the Presence to blur, to let the barrier between your skin and the divine energy around you disappear, and then to let the body and the separation vanish altogether so that you become a centre of consciousness with no barriers and no body. This is an amazing experience and makes you aware of your absolute Oneness with God. It returns you to a state before you entered into the illusion that you were separate from your Divine Source. This will be the subject of the last chapter.

As an aid to this awareness, you might even meditate on the phrase, "I am in you: you are in me," where the "me and you" become interchangeable -- you and God or God and you – you and Abba or Abba and you.

Again, the Bible gives us a little glimpse in story form of what God is to us human beings.

The writers of Genesis explain a profound truth through a simple passage: "In the beginning God created the Heavens and the earth. The earth was without form, and void; and darkness was upon the face of the deep. And the Spirit of God was hovering over the face of the waters. And God said, 'Let there be light: and there was light'" (Genesis 1:1-3).

In this passage, the writer is actually trying to take us to a perception of God beyond words, but he/she has to use words to do that. Usually, we use words to try to describe God and the experience of God but, in the inner path, they often get in the way of understanding. We may say that God is light or love -- which is fine as far as it goes. But in Genesis we see that God creates darkness and the void before light comes into being, even before any order or division arises. At this stage of creation, there are no bodies and only the union of God and the darkness and void.

The darkness and void somehow arise from God, but God is even before the void or darkness. And even though we like to describe God as light, here we see that light is created after darkness and the void. All these words -- darkness, void, light -- that we use to describe God, are words which rightly belong to what has come from God; they cannot express God. The Source from which all comes is what we call, "God."

This is important here in the Silence, because no doctrines or ideas of God can guide us here. Doctrines and words are attempts to give order to our thoughts about God and the world, but here we seek the experience of God, not ideas about God. This is *gnosis*, not *episteme*. In the Silence, we seek experience of the Source, not knowledge about the attributes of God. And remember. The Source is within us.

So we use words metaphorically as Yeshua did in his parables. The words point to the experience of God in our lives, but they do not attempt to define what or who God is. We may say God is like a Father or a Mother or light or love, but all these are things we compare God to because they are things we know, and they give us a sense of familiarity.

The Reality of God is ultimately behind the void and the darkness, behind the light and the love, inexpressible. The Divine experience often involves light and love and joy, but we must not try to dictate how God will come to us or we will put blocks in the way of our spiritual progress.

As the Sages and Saints in many traditions say, we cannot define God with our words and minds: finally, we can only say, "God is in darkness." That may seem like a strange thing to say, but even some of the biblical writers find themselves saying that.

You see, our sense of sight is limited to this world. Our world looks like light and, because light is the most attractive thing to us, we describe God in terms of the most attractive thing. But God is not the light we see with our eyes and we cannot actually see God's ultimate Being which is neither darkness nor light. The Psalmist tries to express this truth when he says, "He made darkness His secret place" (Ps 18:11).

The writers of Genesis also knew this profound truth when they wrote of God being prior to light or darkness, before there were bodies or distinctions, in a state which is a mystery to our senses. The Spirit of God moves upon the chaos of the waters, but God is not the waters themselves.

So, in this quest, we must be humble and not seek to impose our ideas on God, because our ideas will change again and again as we grow spiritually, as we come closer to the Reality of God which Yeshua tells us is within us.

It is good, however, to begin this Practise of the Presence with whatever idea we have of God. We have to start somewhere, and whatever we think of as God, that is the beginning. The experience of the Silence will lead beyond the perception of God as having limits of a particular personality, to the realization of God as beyond any of the limits we might like to impose, including the limits of gender which the English language and many others make it inevitable we use: God IS neither He nor She but we may experience God as He or She.

There is room here, then, for some sense of gender as we humans think of gender. There is a real sense in the experience of the Silence that God does manifest to us in a way that can be thought of as God the Father, "Abba," as Yeshua points out, but also that the Holy Spirit is enfolding and comforting, maternal, the Mother. In Hebrew, the Spirit, *rua*, is feminine and in many traditions, including the early Christian, the Holy Spirit has often been referred to in maternal terms.

So, we will find that, although God as Totality, as the Holy One, cannot be addressed as He or She, the Divine Reality does manifest to us in ways we can relate to our experience of the Father and Mother, the Light and Darkness, the Creative and Destructive, the Life and Death.

According to many of the profound poems in the Bible, we are never apart from God, no matter how negative the experience through which we are going. Thus we read in Psalm 23, "Even though I walk through the Valley of the Shadow of Death, I will fear no evil, For you are with me." Psalm 139 emphasizes this point many times:

> *Where shall I go to escape your Spirit*
>
> *Or where can I flee to escape your Presence?*
>
> *If I ascend into Heaven, you are there:*
>
> *If I make my bed in Sheol [the place of the dead],*
>
> *behold, you are there.*
>
> *If I take the wings of the morning, and dwell in the*
>
> *farthest parts of the sea,*
>
> *Even there will your hand lead me, and your right*
>
> *hand will hold me.*
>
> *If I say, "Surely the darkness will fall on me,"*
>
> *Even the night will be light about me.*
>
> *Yea, the darkness hides not from you:*
>
> *But the night shines as the day:*
>
> *The darkness and the light are both alike to you.*

Like the psalmist, those who have explored these matters extensively know that there is no place and no state of being where we are separate from God.

For our purposes here, that means that we can experience God in any state of our lives. For now it is easiest to have a sense of God's Presence just by feeling that around and within us, in the air we breathe and in the wind that blows, God Is.

Chapter Seven

The Mirror of the Mind: Understanding what is happening in the brain

"In my Father's house are many rooms." (John 14:2)

You know now that the practice of this Prayer of Silence is actually very simple, but it brings you to profound discoveries about your spiritual nature once you know how to do the simple exercises.

With the ideas I have shared and the exercises you have done, you have begun to perceive much about the dynamics of your inner nature. Meditation is at least partly about learning how to develop your "inner senses." The spiritual senses you are developing are aware of inner, spiritual processes which can only be perceived when you close your eyes and concentrate on the things which happen on energy frequencies which are not obvious to the physical senses. You are learning to be aware of what happens inside you as clearly as what happens outside. Yeshua put it this way, "Don't worry so much about washing the outside of the cup: it is the inside of the cup you must clean. It is not what goes into you that defiles you, but what comes out of you. So clean the inside first." (paraphrase of Matt 23:26).

In our everyday living, we usually assume that the only things that are real are the things we can see, touch, smell, taste or hear (although I hope by now you have changed at least some of this attitude from your own experience). Our materialist culture thinks that the things we are doing here in the Silence are merely hallucination caused by being too tired or by being under the influence of drugs or alcohol or some form of mental illness. Sometimes we have nice warm feelings in church or with friends or in a holy place or out in a natural setting, but our culture teaches us that these things are not quite real.

This conflict over what is real and unreal is important to our understanding of what is happening to us as we spend time in the Silence. And, because it is the basis of most of our cultural assumptions, this conflict about the real and the unreal will likely be with you for many years in one form or another as you try to decide what actually is real in your spiritual practice. In order to demonstrate how meditation is actually "real," I thought it might be interesting for you to see what happens to the brain while you meditate. At least that can be considered real, even if much of what we do cannot be measured in physical terms.

An interesting thing which has come out of the scientific study of meditation, using electronic measuring devices, is that it has been discovered that the brain works on different wave lengths, much like a radio or TV, and meditation affects the wave lengths of the brain. It has also been discovered that we pick up certain kinds of sensations on each frequency.

The frequencies have been labelled (from highest frequency to lowest): *gamma, beta, alpha, theta* and *delta.*

Gamma waves are produced when the brain is trying to match two or more sensory modes, as in taste and sound or touch and sight. If you are matching a taste you remember with the sound of a particular tune which was playing at the time you were eating that particular food, your brain is likely producing *gamma* waves which are the highest frequency waves the brain produces (or which have been measured) from 30 to 100 Hz (hertz).

In *beta* consciousness (12 – 30 Hz), the next highest frequency, we carry on our lives as we normally do, shopping, having coffee, eating, talking to others and thinking about where our money and clothes and food are coming from. If we are really tense about things in the world, if we worry a lot or try desperately to think our way out of our problems, we are likely functioning mainly in a high *beta* frequency.

Yeshua tells the people, "Therefore, do not worry about tomorrow, for tomorrow will worry about its own things. Sufficient for the day is its own trouble" (Matt. 6:34). He goes on to say that, instead of worrying, we should "seek first the Kingdom of God and His righteousness" and then the things we need will come when we need them. Note that he is almost telling the people to stop living in *beta* consciousness all the time. It is as if he is saying, "Relax and enter into the lower frequencies where you will find faith and love and peace."

Interestingly, there seems to be little difference in the way the brains of materialists or rigidly religious, moralistic people function. Brain function suggests that a very strict following of religious law may be a form of religious materialism and the brains of materialists may be functioning in *beta* all the time, just like the strictly moralistic people. Yeshua observed this of the Pharisees and the Sadducees who were, respectively, strict moralists and materialists who were trapped in a mechanical way of thinking and would not accept teachings about love, forgiveness, acceptance and the need to come close to God.

If you have this orientation in life or religion, and if your life has become "hard" or "unfeeling," you are likely producing *beta* frequencies most of the time. People who work with mainly *beta* frequencies see immediate benefit from the relaxation exercises in meditation because they have finally found a way to move their brains into the *alpha* frequency.

Beta consciousness, everyday consciousness, is necessary so that we can interact with the world of things, social structures, jobs, difficult people, study, making a living and worrying about tomorrow. When it becomes the only way we think, however, we are only partly what we were designed for as humans.

Unfortunately, a lot of people spend most of their lives in the anxiety, fear, defensiveness and emptiness of pure *beta* consciousness. They develop a sense that the world "out there" is out to get them in some way and they respond to the sense of threat and attack from others with defensiveness and the readiness to attack back with words or deeds. The guns, condemnation and fear of the world come from pure, concentrated, high-grade *beta* consciousness which has never looked beyond itself.

Tense people will often resist entering into the lower frequencies. When they start to meditate, relax and use the lower frequencies of the brain, they may even become frightened, because the lower frequencies uncover a variety of things which they had avoided in life. That is why you were taught to start slowly, with a simple relaxation and a review of the day, so that you did not "burst the old, rigid wineskins." Beyond the rigid view of the world, you have found the more peaceful, loving world which is perceived through the lower frequencies in the brain.

Most of the meditative traditions see *beta* consciousness as a sleep from which we must awake or a darkness from which we must search for the light. *Beta* consciousness is sometimes described as a nightmare of unfulfilled desires, because really, in the material world, all our desires must go unfulfilled: when we do fulfil them, they crumble and disintegrate and we are left with a feeling of emptiness or futility. Remember Alexander the Great crying because there were no more worlds to conquer? That is how we are when we only have material aims and *beta* consciousness.

When you are day-dreaming or when you close your eyes and relax or when you are so absorbed in a relaxed way in some activity that you lose track of what is going on around you, you are likely in "*alpha*" consciousness.

Alpha is a lower frequency of the brain (8 – 12 Hz) and, like a radio receiver, tunes into lower frequency vibrations around you. It is not less real than *beta*; it just notices different types of things. In the same way as *beta* vibrations in you sense the tension of *beta* in others, *alpha* in you will be aware of the *alpha* in others.

Often, *alpha* is called the peaceful brainwave or the spiritual brainwave. That experience of quiet in the church or holy place or watching the sunset on the evening hillside was likely filtered through your *alpha* receptors rather than your other senses. The other senses played a part, but you were picking up other things in the environment that your *beta* senses just can not sense.

You have already used *alpha* consciousness to become aware of some of the peaceful, more spiritual, absorbing things in the world. Entering the Silence on a regular basis will help you to sense those things whenever you want to, because Silence, inner and outer, is one of the fastest ways of tuning into that frequency. What is called the "Relaxation Response" in medical circles is the effect of allowing your brain to slip into *alpha* for a while so the body and brain can heal themselves.

One of the strange ironies of meditation is that *alpha*, which at first seems less in tune with the physical world, actually helps us live more fully in the world. It helps us enjoy life more, see more of what is really going on around us and, by allowing us to draw away from our problems, to consider them in a silent place, it is the ideal way of solving conflict and difficulty.

There are lower frequency waves than *alpha*. *Theta* consciousness (4 – 7 Hz) is associated with what is called hypnagogic imagery, because you are in a deeply relaxed state similar to that produced in hypnotism or self-hypnosis, that strange state that we all experience between sleeping and waking. In that very relaxed state, you tune into things visually -- that is, you see images and pictures in the "mind's eye." (Interestingly, children up to the age of about five often produce *Theta* in their natural level of consciousness and young children often report spiritual experiences or memories of past lives, as if that is the frequency where these things are sensed.)

It is as if, in that state, you can actually see what is in the unconscious mind. You may be able to relive in exact detail events which you had forgotten consciously or you may have a sense that problems you have been trying to solve, work themselves out in symbols before your inner eye.

Sustained *theta* consciousness is usually reached only after quite a lot of practice in meditation, but the problem solving potential or healing potential of *theta* can be achieved quite early in your meditation practice. We will come to that at a later part of our exploration where we use "visualization," which is a form of self-directed hypnagogic imagery, for healing and for creating the alternate world you want.

It might be interesting just for you to speculate on, but the earth's magnetic field resonates at about 7.5 cycles per second (the Schumann resonance), the same frequency as that between the *alpha* and *theta* range in the human brain. Could it be that in entering the *theta*/low *alpha* frequencies, we are coming into harmony with many of the complex forces which make up our living earth? Our bodies are made from the earth and return to the earth: the state of our world indicates that we really do need to get in tune with our earth, so just for the sake of our health and the health of our world, entering regularly into the Silence is a great benefit.

Researchers have also found that we enter the *theta* range when we are actively seeking to resolve things from our subconscious mind. It is as if many things which we have repressed are stored out of reach of our usual awareness, but when we really want to get in touch with them, we can do so by slowing down the brain waves so that these things can emerge. We will use that healing potential often in the exercises which follow.

Regular meditation will make it easier to move into the lower frequencies and heal what is there. This is likely also the reason why we may be able to resolve a particular issue, only to have the same issue come up ten years later. Different aspects of the issue have been stored in lower frequencies in the brain and only when we can enter that frequency can we heal it. This is likely for our own protection, so that the really traumatic memories will not overwhelm us until we have done enough meditation to be able to address them.

Beta is valuable because it helps us to focus narrowly, to deal with life's many challenges with a sense of immediacy, and to work out problems in a concentrated, intellectually focussed way. *Beta* is part of us and should not be denied. However, it should not be the only part of our mental abilities we use. *Alpha* and lower frequencies help us see things in a wider context so that we do not get trapped into the narrowness of *beta*. What we call "narrow minded people" may actually be operating on a very narrow wave band: meditation helps widen that band to communicate more fully.

Delta consciousness, the lowest frequency (up to 4 Hz), is common in children and is what we produce in sleep. Until recently, experimenters thought that was all it was for. Just recently (2009) I heard a commentator on television saying that if you are producing *delta* it means you are almost dead! This is not the case. With more sophisticated equipment, researchers have discovered that *delta* is in use while we are awake as well. When the brain is producing *delta* waves, however, it seems the mind is searching in the widest possible way for solutions or information. If I ask you to "Quote your favourite line of poetry," and you do not know the answer immediately, but have to search in your mind over all the poems you have ever heard, you are likely producing *delta*. You may also be using *delta* to deal with repressed trauma, especially if what you are dealing with requires that you search widely in all your experience for answers to the questions you have to deal with.

People are capable of communicating with each other, often over great distances, by some psychic/spiritual means. Most families have stories about this kind of communication and many people have experienced it in some form. Psychologists researching this area call it "para-psychology" or "Transpersonal Psychology" because in this type of psychology it is not just your own psychological states that are involved: they extend between persons or into what is beyond conventional psychology. It is likely that the very low frequency vibrations are involved in maintaining the connections between us at levels we are not usually aware of,

People with psychic and healing abilities seem to produce more *theta* while they are going about their daily business. Their brains seem to be permanently tuned into the lower frequencies. The other side of that is true as well: as you learn to meditate and your brain moves into lower frequencies, you will produce *theta* and *delta* more readily and you will very often have psychic and mystic experiences.

The names *gamma, beta, alpha, theta* and *delta* are just arbitrary names given by researchers to different brain frequencies. However, beyond the scientific terminology, which helps us to visualize in a simplified form what is happening in the brain as it enters higher or lower frequencies, this whole matter is really a way of saying that we are potentially conscious on more than one level, in the same way as a television can pick up signals on different frequencies.

I am not aware of any research into brain waves and what we call wisdom, but I would suspect that the wise person is using more of the lower frequencies and also all of the frequencies at the same time, in order to process more types of information before coming to a conclusion. If that is the case, then practicing *the Prayer of Silence* should make you wise.

We are not just physical bodies sensing physical objects. We are actually capable of entering into much more complex relations with others, with the universe and with the Divine than appears to our untrained senses. In *the Prayer of Silence* we are training our inner senses gradually to enter the lower frequencies which perceive more and more subtle and inclusive things about life.

With all this talk of the brain, it is important to emphasize that our consciousness is not confined to the brain. You have already begun to experience much non-brain awareness. But reviewing the brain's various functions gives us a brief glimpse of some of what is happening to us spiritually, beyond the brain. As you meditate, you now know that you are activating a larger part of your mental and spiritual capacity than when you are not meditating. You can actually train your consciousness to be aware of deeper and more profound realities as the years go by.

Studying the brain and its relationship to consciousness also confirms something we have spoken of before. We have already quoted Yeshua's warning, "Do not put new wine in old wineskins or they will burst and the wine will be spilled." Brain research indicates that this is actually good advice for mental health.

It is known now that the gateway to the spiritual dimensions is in the lower frequencies of the brain, in *alpha*, *theta* and *delta*. People with advanced spiritual experience produce these waves regularly in their everyday lives and in their meditative states. It is also known that repressed negative memories are also stored in *theta* and perhaps also in *delta*. People who are trying to resolve a lot of repressed material also produce high amplitude *theta* and *delta*. In this phenomenon we get a little glimpse of what is happening to the brain as we struggle with the darkness within us and then as we live creatively beyond the resolved conflicts.

Many spiritual traditions teach that there are dragons, lions or other monsters or terrifying angels protecting the higher spiritual levels or the higher Heavens. They say that if you continue on the spiritual path you will encounter these monsters and will have to defeat them before you can proceed farther.

Likewise, we know that, when you encounter repressed material in the brain in the *theta* level, it often appears in symbolic, terrifying form. *Theta* awareness tends to see things symbolically rather than literally. And we also know that, as you move your consciousness into the lower frequencies, where the spiritual perceptions exist, you also have to encounter and resolve all the repressed memories and fears before you can go very far in that direction. So the spiritual traditions and the study of brain frequencies say the same thing – that when we get into the deeper spiritual states we have to face the dragons of the mind in order to progress further.

For our own sakes, then, we must change gradually and meditate without looking for the "quick fix," in order not to strain the old wineskins, our old habits of thinking and reacting, and in order not to get into the repressed content in the brain too quickly. (Later chapters present a number of ways of entering gradually and safely into that darkness.)

A few examples might help to understand what is involved in "meeting the dragons" of the mind on the road to wholeness.

A student once came to me and said that every time she tried to write an essay she became very frightened (writing is a creative process which draws on the lower frequencies of the brain to integrate ideas and insights, so she was entering into the lower frequencies of the brain in trying to write but was also faced with repressed material at the same time). After some discussion, I asked her to close her eyes, relax and tell me what it felt like to have the fear of writing. She almost immediately entered into the material stored in the *theta* frequencies of her brain and became very frightened. What she saw in her "mind's eye" was a great monster trying to attack her. I asked her to surround herself with light and then to let the monster of the mind attack to see what would happen. I told her it was of the mind and could not hurt her.

She relaxed and surrounded herself with light and then let the monster attack. After this, I saw her visibly relax. She recounted that the monster had disappeared and her Grade Five classroom came into her mind. There she could see herself as a little girl reading her essay before the class and every time she made a mistake the teacher hit her with a ruler. She had forgotten the incident but the fear itself had become a monster for her. After we explored and discussed that experience for a bit, she had no more difficulty writing essays.

Notice that after she was able to deal with the repressed memory, which was stored in *theta*, she was able to use the creative potential of *theta* to write her essays from then on. The frightening memory was acting as a monster blocking access to her creativity.

Someone I know started a meditative prayer group in his home Baptist church. He started by asking the group just to sit quietly for three minutes with eyes closed. Most of the members of the group found it very relaxing, no more, but three members got up and left angrily. They reported to the minister that they were being taught devil worship -- in those three minutes of silence they had seen in themselves the tremendous fear of evil and the devil that was just under the surface of their consciousness. They were not being taught devil worship: they were merely discovering how close their obsession with the devil and evil was to the surface of their minds.

Again, if they had been able to confront the fear in their minds, they would have been able to move on to the creative and healing potential of meditation.

William Blake says that those who never change their ideas "are like standing water and breed monsters of the mind." The three members of that group, the student afraid of essays and most of us are like the stagnant water, and we may run into the monsters in our minds very quickly.

But, as Carl Jung says, we must face the "shadow" in ourselves, or "meet our personal devils" in order to become whole, in the same way Yeshua had to meet his Satan in the wilderness. (In Jewish writing "the Satan" is always the adversary, the angel sent by God to provide testing and to see if the hero is ready to proceed farther on the spiritual path, as in the book of Job in the Old Testament.) By "meeting our personal devil," Jung meant that we have to look at the darker side of ourselves, know what really could tempt us and then come to terms with that part of ourselves in order to move on to the creativity which is blocked by the negative memories or attitudes or beliefs. The dark side of our nature can be frightening, especially if we come upon it without adequate preparation and in the symbolic form which *theta* consciousness provides. Once we have faced it, like the girl afraid of essays, we are free to go on to more constructive living.

Another woman in a meditation group came to me after the first session and said she thought I could help her. Her problems seemed very daunting once she outlined them. She had been to see psychiatrists, she said, and doctors and had been on anti-psychotic drugs but still, every time she closed her eyes, all she saw was a black and frightening devil which wanted to steal her soul. After some discussion I got her to do the same as the woman with the fear of essays – I asked her to relax, surround herself with light, ask for divine protection and then to allow the devil (who stood menacingly in her mind) to attack her.

As soon as she allowed the devil to attack, it disappeared and never returned. She did not have to use anti-psychotic drugs after that. However, releasing the fear which had kept the devil in place for so many years, also allowed her to explore the reasons for the symbolic devil being there. She had been raised a Roman Catholic but in a family in which almost all the children were sexually abused. As an adult, she had been raped while working overseas and had then had an abortion, for which her family and her priest condemned her, telling her she would go to Hell. Her mind had stored all of this material, including the religious beliefs with which she had been raised, in *theta* and had transformed it into the symbol of the devil which was trying to steal her soul. It was fear which fed the symbolic devil. Once she let go of the fear, the devil disappeared and she was then able to deal creatively with the rest of the repressed content from her childhood and later adulthood.

Notice how the ancient traditions of the dragons and monsters guarding the advanced levels of spiritual functioning are actually based on what really happens as we try to grow spiritually. *Theta* produces symbols which speak to us of the darker experiences we have repressed. These symbols tell us what we have to overcome if we are to progress further. And once we deal with the symbolic guardians, we are wise enough to go on into the more advanced levels of spiritual development.

Theta's use of symbols is also very useful in the visualization and healing exercises I will teach you shortly. Once we deal with the negative aspects of what we have stored in *theta*, we can use the tremendously powerful healing and creative aspects of the level of consciousness which can be measured as *theta*, to heal mind, body, emotions and relationships. *Theta* can also be used to enhance the creativity of artists, inventors, scientists, musicians and other people who create new things and ideas. Combined with the Watcher perspective, it is a tremendously powerful agent of transformation.

The brain is structured in such a way that it gives rise to different kinds of meaning depending on which part of the brain is used. The left brain is logical and mathematical. It takes one thing at a time to draw its conclusions logically. When the left brain and *beta* consciousness are combined we have a powerful problem solving organ.

The right brain tends to see patterns and to see meaning in holistic terms, not just in a series of logical steps. The right brain tends to be more intuitive and creative. That process is accentuated by *alpha* and *theta* consciousness to see deeper, relaxed meaning in things or to resolve complex problems and seek balance.

Meditation tends to move us toward *alpha* and *theta* but also toward right brain knowledge. There is an actual brain basis for the division between epistemological (left brain, *beta*) and gnostic (right brain, *alpha* and *theta*) knowing. We can see in brain terms why Yeshua taught in parables, stories with patterns which force us to think with the right brain and with *alpha* and *theta* consciousness instead of with left brain, *beta* consciousness. He wanted people to look more deeply at the meaning of their lives.

The brain is part of the body, but we now know from experience that our bodies and brains are not just physical things without spirit. We are actually hard-wired, as they say, for spiritual perception. Meditation trains us to do things for which we were designed from the beginning. The brain is a spiritual "machine."

If the brain is a computer, as some people argue, then it is a computer which was designed from the beginning to lead us to spiritual perception. Researchers have often commented on the "excess capacity" which is built into the brain. We only use about 5% of our potential brain resources, and researchers have only recently discovered that the brain can grow more capacity when it is needed. This is called "brain plasticity." Why do we have all this extra, unused capacity?

From brain studies with people who have done a lot of meditation, it would appear that there is great potential for spiritual perception which we are only starting to use. This excess capacity cannot be the result of "evolutionary pressures," which is what is usually presented as the cause of our physical characteristics. Instead, it appears that the brain is an organ of perception which is waiting for something which the "designer" knew we would use some time in the future, but for which we have not been ready until now. That means the cause of the structure of the brain is actually in the future, and its fulfilment will come as we continue to explore more of our spiritual potential over time.

There are amazingly positive things available in the Silence, and brain research is only beginning to scratch the surface of what can be achieved through meditation. Once we deal with the darkness in ourselves, with the repressed memories in *theta*, we open huge potential for creativity, for co-operation, for Love, Joy and Peace "which pass all understanding," as Yeshua says.

It is one of the challenges and joys of this way of Inner Silence that there is a larger world to move into. We are not as limited as we usually think we are. Or as Yeshua says, "In my Father's house are many rooms." There is much potential there to explore.

All of the exercises we have done have moved us beyond the ordinary world we lived in before we started on this way of Silence. In brain terms, we have started the long journey from the higher frequencies, which see only the insistent, tension filled activity of every day, to the lower frequencies, which can perceive and resolve the negative things which keep us tied to our fears. That opens the creative and peace filled frequencies so that we can manifest the Kingdom of God on earth as it is in Heaven.

Notice that these changes are not caused by the brain. The brain is not the source of this elevated consciousness. Using the Watcher, which is outside the physical body, we have actually willed changes in the brain. It is our non-brain consciousness which has made it possible for the brain to change and accommodate our vision of what we want to be.

We are re-establishing a connection with our deeper spiritual nature, and with God, which has been broken, for most people, for quite some time. Or as St. Paul puts it, "For now we see in a mirror, dimly, but then face to face. Now I know in part, but then I shall know just as I also am known" (I Cor 13:12).

That face to face encounter with God and with ourselves is what we seek and what we can achieve with devotion and trust, and brain research confirms what the great spiritual traditions have known for centuries – that we are not slaves of the body and the brain but we are capable of initiating spiritual growth from within ourselves, which in turn can change the body and the brain.

Chapter Eight

The Mystery of the Body

*"Do you not know that you are the temple of God,
and that the Spirit of God dwells in you?" (I Cor. 3:16)*

There is a strange irony about this opening quotation. It can be taken literally, in saying that God lives in us, only when we understand the body through the eyes of science, and when we do that, we discover some very interesting things about the nature of the body, of consciousness, of healing and of what we are doing in the Prayer of Silence.

The body holds a great spiritual mystery, but bodies are troublesome and, in consequence, most "spiritual" people do not like bodies and the things that bodies do. Spiritual disciplines often prescribe a variety of ways to "subdue the body," to cover it up with clothes, beat it into submission, starve it, punish it with self-inflicted pain or ignore it completely. Many meditative traditions are designed to repress the body and its urges. Some traditions go so far as to say that the body is evil or even that the body is the cause of all evil.

Admittedly, the body does have a number of things against it. It gets hungry and thirsty, it is sometimes stinky, it is involved in defecation and sex, it decays at death (and sometimes before death) and it tends to get sick and old. The body can be quite ugly and it usually seeks its own comfort and survival instead of being concerned with others. The body reminds us that we are animals. It seems to give rise to things like lust and gluttony and other desires which can imprison us. So, in order to be holy, many traditions prescribe fasting, abstaining from sex and food or causing the body discomfort, even pain, in order to force the attention onto more "spiritual" matters.

This bias against the body comes from the belief that the "spirit" is somehow opposite to or opposed to the body. From this belief comes the pledge in some churches to "renounce the world, the flesh and the devil," as if the flesh is the same as the devil. However, as in many other things, Yeshua challenged these notions directly, and in the Prayer of Silence, taking our lead from him, we make the body the centre of a great deal of our meditation.

Yeshua spoke of the body differently: "The lamp of the body is the eye. If therefore your eye is good, your whole body will be full of light. But if your eye is bad, your whole body will be full of darkness" (Matt 6:22-23). In this passage, he says that the body is neither good nor bad. It is the "eye," the way we see things, which is good or bad.

Yeshua makes the same point in another parable taken from everyday life -- washing the dishes after eating: "For you cleanse the outside of the cup and dish, but inside they are full of extortion and self-indulgence. . . . first cleanse the inside of the cup and dish, that the outside of them may be clean also" (Matt. 23:25-26). When you condemn the body, he is saying, it is as ridiculous as condemning the cup for being unclean. The cup and dish are neither good nor bad; they are only dirty if you do not clean them. The parable means that the body does not cause lust and greed and gluttony. These come from within.

The Prayer of Silence is a spiritual discipline which sees the body as a clue to the mystery of our spiritual condition. So we spend a lot of time looking inside the body to see if it has been "washed properly," not trying to avoid it.

***

Meditation Exercise: Practising contemplation

I spent most of my career as a university professor, teaching people how to think. I am doing the same thing here, except I am teaching you how to think differently than most people are used to. One of the ways to create "new knowledge" is through contemplation – looking in meditation at the implications of ideas. This is the creative use of consciousness, the kind which great scientists, writers, philosophers and artists use, where the mind itself is encouraged to create new ideas, theories and visions.

Yeshua tells us we need to clean up our ideas and attitudes, the way we "see" things. In order to do that we need to focus some of our attention on what our ideas imply about us. We need to examine "the inside of the cup." Without that focus we cannot grow spiritually.

In the exercises so far, we have been exploring our actions and our world from the perspective of the Watcher. We have become aware of how God can be perceived in the world around us. But we have so far stayed away from concentrating on ideas themselves in our meditation, even if ideas have come up indirectly, in the discussions between exercises. The focus has been mainly on our actions, emotions, memories, attitudes and awareness of the world.

We will now add to this focus by moving our attention to an awareness of the ideas in the mind. In order to clarify the meanings of the subjects we are exploring in these pages, it would be good, as part of your practise of entering the Silence, to explore some of the ideas I talk about here. You will then be able to carry over this kind of exploration of implications of ideas into other areas of your thinking life. You can contemplate on any ideas from any of your reading or from various media. Spiritual growth is often aided by contemplation on passages from the Scriptures so that you see the deeper meanings which are hidden from a cursory reading.

Meditating on ideas is called "contemplation." It involves bringing ideas into your time in the Silence, asking God's guidance to find out what they have to say to you in your situation, and then observing from the Watcher's perspective while the meaning unfolds before you. Often, the meaning will not be in words at all, but in a growing awareness, almost like looking at an abstract pattern of meaning arising around you.

Remember how *theta* consciousness tends to transform things into symbols and the right brain translates things into patterns instead of logical, step by step arguments? Often, when you contemplate on ideas, the relaxed attention of meditation will take you into *theta* brain function, and *theta* will translate those ideas into symbols for you to understand, or will create visual images which will help you appreciate the full meaning of the ideas.

You do not have to wait till the morning or evening to do this exercise. Many times you will be confronted with an idea during the day and will not want to wait to explore its meaning. This exercise should be done whenever you are faced with an idea, often while reading or listening to a lecture or the TV. You can do "meditative reading" by stopping whenever needed, closing your eyes, entering quickly into the Silence, and observing in your mind how the ideas you have just read or heard are transformed by a deeper meditative exploration.

You do not need to agree with the ideas, as long as you explore and clarify them for yourself. Do not use a lot of words in your contemplation of ideas.

That will only confine you to *beta* consciousness. Like the other meditations, this one is not for developing logical arguments to have with someone else: contemplation gives you a sense of "awareness" of the deeper meaning of the ideas for you and your life. You will find, as you bring ideas into your time in the Silence, that ideas have a shape and texture of their own. They are visual and can be seen as patterns. When you contemplate, you turn the epistemological knowledge into your own *gnosis* – you make it your own.

You may wonder why I say we are going to concentrate on the mystery of the body and then say we are going to focus on ideas. That is because ***our ideas about the body (or about anything else) actually affect how we see the body***. If you have been taught that the body is bad, you will look for all the bad things in the body. If you have learned that the body is just material substance with no spiritual meaning, that is what you will see, and you will judge the body as ultimately meaningless because it is "just matter."

In this chapter, we focus on ideas about the mystery of the body. It is fairly easy to bring ideas about the body into contemplation because the body is "physical" and has shape and substance. You can visualize any of the things I talk about. Feet and hands and ears are easy to visualize. Perhaps more difficult are cells, energy fields, DNA double helix, sunshine, sub-atomic particles and other things of that sort, but they can be brought into your meditation as "pictures in the mind" as well. It will help you to understand what I am saying if you can stop once in a while and visualize what I am saying about the body.

Contemplation will also help develop an aspect of the mind which most people ignore. There are actually two minds in us. There is the mind which is very logical and uses a lot of words to develop coherent arguments, one step at a time. This "mind" is actually centred in the left side of the brain, as we have seen.

Then there is another mind, centred in the right brain, which sees relationships and patterns and is open to creativity, insight, intuition and other kinds of knowing which see, not in individual, separated bits, but with a greater sense of unity and connection.

Both sides of the brain are connected by something called the *corpus callosum*. It is a bundle of connective neural structures which make communication between the right and left hemispheres possible. In the same way as both sides of the brain are necessary, so too both kinds of thinking are important and necessary. If you contemplate on this paragraph, for instance, you will find that it is structured to emphasize, in all its elements, the parallel between the brain structure, knowledge and words. *Beta* and left brain consciousness is reflected in it, because it is made up of a logical sequence of ideas, held together with logical words or phrases like, "for instance," "in the same way as," "so too," "both. . . are necessary," "for instance," "like." It also contains a pattern, which is right brain/ *theta* function – with a contrast between two ways of seeing, connected to two types of brain function, with connective "tissue" of words providing the link between them. To contemplate on this paragraph would involve visualizing the two sides of the brain along with the connecting *corpus callosum,* and then visualizing how the different brain functions, the different brain wave patterns and the different types of thinking are related to this physical structure.

If you do not know anything about the brain (or whatever else we are discussing) it might help to check on the internet or in the library for information about the brain so that you can accurately visualize what is going on. Contemplation often involves checking information to see if it is accurate. Much of the research which people conduct in libraries or laboratories is actually a form of contemplation. In doing my own academic research on the literature of the world, for instance, I have spent years in careful contemplation of the implications of what I read.

This exercise is not a short one which stops anywhere. It will be a continuing exercise which, like the awareness of everyday activity around you, will help you grow in "mind knowledge" in a deeper way for the rest of your life, as you train yourself to see the "mind patterns" which are important for your spiritual growth. Spiritual evolution cannot proceed by suppressing ideas: it must incorporate ideas as part of the developing total awareness of your being.

Almost all spiritual traditions advise us to spend time in study and learning. In Hindu Yoga there is a whole branch of the discipline, called *Jnana Yoga,* which is devoted to learning and contemplation, so that one may come to the realization of "correct knowledge" which can lead to the equivalent of *Gnosis*, the knowledge of oneness with God. Ignorance is one of the greatest obstacles to enlightenment.

***

What follows in the rest of this chapter will require that you do a lot of contemplation in order to understand all the implications of what I present to you about the body and its underlying mystery. You can use my words as the basis for contemplation, to clarify your idea of what the body is. You do not have to agree with me. These ideas are presented as an aid to your own under-standing. As you read, see if you can visualize the things I write about. Since I am writing about the body, try to sense in your own body, the implications of what I say.

The body, unlike the nebulous "spirit," is quite obvious to us. It is some-thing of which we are all too painfully aware, from the time we take our first breath or start to grow out first teeth to when we (or rather, our bodies) die. We know now that we never die.

The body is especially troublesome when it decides to malfunction. We seem so obviously to be bodies, in fact, that it is often hard to think of our-selves as spiritual at all. Some people think that it is even misleading to speak of the "spirit" -- we are really only bodies and nothing more, they claim.

One of the basic principles of the Prayer of Silence is that we are whole beings and consist of a number of aspects -- body, spirit, emotions, mind and life energy all functioning together.

Another principle which arises from approaching life as a unity is that we can always get anywhere else from where we are now. Any aspect of our ex-istence can be an avenue into an experience of other aspects of our wholeness. We can, therefore, get to know our spiritual being through our bodies, or our bodies through our emotions, or our emotions through our minds, and so on. As we contemplate any one principle in ourselves, we end up connecting with the meaning of all the other principles.

Another of the operating ideas of the Prayer of Silence is that we (includ-ing our bodies) arise from what we have called pure Spirit, Atman, *Christos*, the Ray of the Divine Light. We have moved away from our Source, but we are finding our way back to awareness of that spiritual origin.

Yeshua has a metaphor directly related to our origin in God and our con-tinuing relationship to our Divine Source: "I am the true vine, and My Father is the vinedresser. Every branch in Me that does not bear fruit He takes away; and every branch that bears fruit He prunes, that it may bear more fruit" (John 15:1-2). Notice the phrase, "in Me." This is not a parable about the wicked being punished, as many people say. It is a parable about spiritual growth. In the spiritual life, the choices we make which do not bear good fruit can always be corrected by pruning as we commune with God, so that the fruitful choices can cause more productive growth.

To turn the above paragraph (or any of Yeshua's parables) into a contemplation exercise, re-read the passage, become aware of the patterns in it, close your eyes, relax, ask for guidance and then, from the perspective of the Watcher, bring the patterns of ideas into your mind. Visualize the vine and what the story says about the vine.

Yeshua has branches which God prunes. What are the branches? Abilities? Ideas? Actions? Perhaps we are some of his branches. If we are like Yeshua, we also have branches. If our branches do not bear fruit, they are pruned. Pruning branches on vines makes the vine bear more fruit. Visualize the pruning and what that achieves in you and in Yeshua. If Yeshua is the true vine, where are his roots? Where are our roots? Continue to visualize what is in the passage and then allow any connections "to make themselves" as you allow your spirit to speak to you. What does the parable say about your own nature? If this is a *koan*, what does it tell you about spiritual enlightenment?

When you have finished that process, you have made the understanding of the parable your own. You have developed an inner understanding on which you can build in the future.

In order to write this book, I had to go through all of its ideas in this way, allowing the ideas to develop and grow until I saw their larger implications for the spiritual life. The ideas grew in me while I was in the Silence of God.

The parable above does not mention the roots, but when I read the parable, I immediately think of those un-named roots. Yeshua is the vine but where are his roots? Roots usually involve origins. What are our origins? It seems to me that by leaving out the roots, Yeshua was actually calling our attention to them by their omission, since roots are one of the most important parts of a plant. Contemplation brings our attention to that part of the story, whereas people looking for literal meanings would not even bother to think about that.

As I think about the roots I wonder, "How does the Torah, the Jewish scripture, envisage our origins?" This is a valid question, since Yeshua drew most of his teachings from the Torah. In a primary way, the Torah says, our origins are explained in the first chapter of Genesis. That takes us back to, "In the beginning," since we are in the image of God. In the beginning, we arose from God. In the beginning was even before the Void and the Darkness were brought into being, and certainly before the world existed.

In the modern world we tend to think that our beginning was somewhere in the ancient, pre-historic world, before we evolved from early life forms.

But the Torah says that God is our Source, not anything in the world. That is as far back as we can get.

But that is going very far back. More immediately, like the vine growing, we continually arise, individually, from day to day, from something else. All our cells change, continually, but we remain essentially the same person. Where do we come from each day? Here my contemplation tells me there is a connection between the biblical account and some very interesting modern discoveries.

Theoretical physicists tell us that our bodies are changing all the time. Every atom and sub-atomic particle is continually coming into being and vanishing. We seem to be arising continually from what is called the "Zero Point Field." If you could remove all the matter and energy from a particular space, you would still have something which physicists call the Zero Point Field. You would not be left with nothing, if you removed everything. You would still have the Zero Point Field which is still full of some kind of undefined activity – an activity without matter or energy, which seems to be a contradiction. Classical physics teaches that there is only matter and energy in the universe, and that if you remove matter and energy, you have a nothing left. But the Zero Point Field is obviously not nothing. The trouble is, no one knows what it is. Some scientists think this activity in the realm beyond matter and energy may be consciousness.

There seems to be a parallel between this Zero Point Field and what John's Gospel calls the "Light that lights every person coming into the world." He also refers to this Light as the *Logos*. The *Logos* is the primary being from which the universe arises. John says that it was through the *Logos* that the universe came into being. Calling the Source, "*Logos*," is another way of saying "God," but *Logos* was and is an active force, because the universe continually arises from this "God force." It is the Source of all that is.

This *Logos* Light is the root from which all comes. It is ultimately the root of the vine Yeshua spoke of in his parable of the vine. And the *Logos* is almost like the Zero Point Field from which everything seems to arise, continually. Some physicists even speak of the Zero Point Field as the mind of God. Somehow this field, just like the *Logos*, is the source of our being, continually, all the time manifesting the physical body which we think of as "us." If this is true, our bodies are not just matter. They are the expression of a constant creative process which is taking place all over the universe, all the time.

However, as our bodies come into being every instant, they reflect our ideas and attitudes and feelings. If we have negative feelings about ourselves, these feelings are manifest in our bodies. If we think positively about ourselves, these feelings are manifest in our bodies.

Somehow our consciousness seems to be related to the Zero Point Field, the Mind of God, in that our consciousness determines much of what manifests as our body. That is an oversimplification, of course, because there are an almost infinite number of forces at work in manifesting who we are, but it does indicate that, if we look closely at our bodies, we can actually see the results of our emotions, our ideas and our spiritual nature.

That means that our bodies are very important, because they tell us the kinds of energies which have produced this physical expression we call "body."

In the spiritual tradition within which I am a student and teacher, it is very important to distinguish between "creation" and "manifestation." We tend to speak of God "creating" the universe. By using that word, we automatically distance God from the universe, with God somehow tinkering with the universe like a man fixing a car. In that tradition, the universe is seen as something mechanical and separate from God.

The tradition reflected in *the Prayer of Silence* speaks of the "manifestation," rather than the "creation," of the universe. That is an important distinction. There is no separation between God and the universe in this view, because the universe includes in itself the nature and presence of God. The reason we have consciousness is not because God somehow "made" us to have consciousness. Rather, God's nature is consciousness, and being in the image of God, we also have consciousness. In fact, our consciousness is inseparable from God's consciousness. In this sense, Atman/Spirit and God are one, in the same way that a drop of water and the ocean are one. Atman/Spirit is in everything as a direct expression of God, so that, as Yeshua says, "But the very hairs of your head are all numbered" (Matt 10:30). The implication of this statement is that God is present, not just in your body, but in each hair and in each sparrow and each blade of grass.

Think of God, not as separate from "the creation," but rather as "the consciousness of the manifested universe." When you speak to God in meditation, then, you are communicating directly from your consciousness with the consciousness of the universe -- from the drop to the ocean. There is no distance, no separation between the drop and the ocean. In advanced stages of meditation, your consciousness and the consciousness of the universe become one and, like Yeshua, you know, "I and My Father are one."

This is an ideal subject for contemplation because there is a parallel operating here. Allow these ideas to enter into your time in the Silence. Actually feel the way the ideas are related to each other. Feel the patterns of the ideas and how they are related to your own experience of the world and of the Silence.

Mystical philosophers often say, "As above, so below." In this phrase is summed up a profound realization about the relationship between God and humanity. In the same way you and I have a body which is animated by consciousness, so too, the universe is a body and God is the consciousness of that body. "Above," which means in the divine sphere, the universe is body and God is consciousness. "Below," which means in the human sphere, we have a body of which we are the consciousness – the corresponding pattern which is found in the divine scheme of things, is also found in the human scheme because we are a manifestation of the very nature of God.

We know from experience that there is some aspect of our being which is more profoundly "us" than an arm or a leg. If you remove our arms and legs we are still "me" in some way. The question is, how much do you have to trim away before you come to the "me" at the centre?

The Prayer of Silence demonstrates that the most fundamental "me" I can arrive at, after all else is stripped away, is Atman/Spirit, as we explored earlier in this book, and that this Atman/Spirit is very directly an expression, a "manifestation" of God's Spirit. Because we arise from Divine Spirit, in our most profound awareness of the deepest aspects of ourselves, we are experiencing this Divine Spirit. The Spirit within us is, as the Jewish writers say, a Spark of the Divine Fire. When we find the answer to the question, "Who am I?" we will know the answer to the question, "Who is God?"

There are difficulties here, however. We cannot start removing limbs to find out what is left. We are in bodies and we have to function with our bodies and take them seriously -- not as separate from Spirit, but as aspects of Spirit. The body is that aspect of Spirit which we can perceive with the senses.

This approach to the relationship between God and humanity, the one which sees the body as the temple of God, is very different from most Christian, Jewish and Islamic traditions. In those, God is completely separate from "the creation." The Jewish philosopher, Martin Buber, expresses this separation by saying that the relationship between human beings and God is like that between "I and Thou." In the "I and Thou" relationship, there is always an absolute separation, always the sense that we and God are separate "persons." Yeshua, on the other hand, said, "I and My Father are One," "the Kingdom of God is within you," the Kingdom of God, the Presence of God is like salt which gives flavour to your being. There is no separation between us and God as the origin of our being.

How is consciousness related to the universe, then? Is the universe just dead matter, as the materialist scientific tradition suggests? In the Prayer of Silence we say that consciousness is latent within all parts of the universe, even in the rocks, because the universe is a manifestation of God. Time allows that latent quality of consciousness to manifest itself, because time also is an aspect of the divine unfolding of the universe.

Some people will pounce at this point (as they have in discussions) and say, "Ah ha! You are a pantheist. You believe that the universe is God."

To which I replay, "No. The universe is not God. However, nothing can be separate from God. If God is the Source of all that is, then nothing can have had any other source. The whole universe must be a manifestation of some of what God is -- although it cannot be God, or God is no longer Source."

It is important to make that distinction. The totality of what God is cannot be known but, in the universe, we can see some of what God is because the universe reflects the nature of God, the Source of "All that Is." Therefore, when we trace back the origins of the body (or rocks or trees) to the beginning, we will ultimately find consciousness and God.

"Why is all of this abstraction important?" you may ask.

Our present culture is primarily materialist. It argues that there are really only material things, and that consciousness is merely an aberration, what is called in scientific terms, "epiphenomenal," something which is merely an added, superficial feature of physical phenomena, like froth on a wave. The wave is the "real" thing, they argue: the froth is merely something else which arises from the action of the wave. In the materialist's view, meditation is even more "frothy" than ordinary consciousness because, when we enter the Silence, we still the action of our material body (like stilling the wave) and so anything which arises from that stillness is even further away from the material base of existence and hence less real.

In order to counter this argument of the materialists, we have actually experienced that consciousness is primary. It does not arise from the material world as something added, like froth, but it is the basis from which all else arises. Consciousness, like the Zero Point Field, and not material substance, is the primary reality, and meditation puts us in contact with that primary, causal reality.

It is also important to establish that we and God are one because, in most of the monotheistic religious traditions, meditation on our inner being is seen as meaningless, because they teach that God is outside us and our world and that we are really only supposed to try to please God by obeying God's command-ments and believing the right doctrines. The aim of the spiritual life in most of these traditions is to get into Heaven or Paradise and avoid Hell. If we can believe rightly and act properly, they say, then we can get into Heaven. These traditions usually portray God as a personality somehow set over against us, separate from us and separate from the world. God is seen as the "Creator," and we and the world are the "creatures." Prayer is merely a way of trying to make contact with "the God at a distance."

But Yeshua tells us that we and God are one, that it is possible to find God within our own consciousness, because the consciousness of God and our con-sciousness are one. He also says this in parable form where God is the root of the vine, Yeshua is the vine and we are the branches but we all have our roots in God. All are interconnected without separation.

The Prayer of Silence is based on the great mystery of the body, which is summarized in the biblical claim that the body is the temple of God. When we truly know the body, we can know God, not because the body is itself God, but because the body manifests some of the essential consciousness of God with which we seek union.

***

This takes us to another question which is very important in our present materialist age: What is the body? Is it a machine, a bunch of organs, base matter, dust and ashes, a complex chemical soup? Or is there something more to it, as Yeshua taught?

Ironically, modern science, which is officially a materialist approach to exploring the universe, presents us with some interesting clues. I will pres-ent you with three stories of scientific discoveries about the nature of bodies which will illustrate what I mean when I say that God is the consciousness of the universe.

I was waiting for a doctor's appointment and picked up a medical journal. Much to my surprise I discovered something very important about the nature of bodies. The human body (and all living things) are made up of cells. At the heart of each cell is the DNA double helix molecule, like a long spiral staircase with three billion steps in each molecule. Each step is made up of a pair of chemicals called "nucleotides." This chemical pair is very powerful because it controls everything from the colour of your hair to the shape of your nose and the size of your liver. No two people have the same DNA, which is why DNA has become so important in court cases, to identify the culprit in a crime.

Each of the steps of the DNA "staircase" is given a combination of numbers and letters in order to map the human genome. If you listed all the numbers/letters of the chemical pairs in telephone books, and then stacked the phone books one on top of the other, you would have a stack of books as high as a fifty-five story building! Yet all of that information, encoded in chemical pairs, is stored as only a small part of every cell in every living thing on the planet. Imagine the number of telephone book it would take to map all the chemical pairs in all the cells of all the living organisms on earth.

One small error in copying the chemical information when the cell divides, causes large changes in the body. It might even cause disease or death. Remember, there are about three billion steps in every DNA double helix in every cell in the body. It is estimated that in each human body there are from 50 to 75 trillion cells. Each one of these cells has a specific function, not only in terms of the immediate environment of the organ or other system in which it exists, but also in relation to the whole of the body. Everything exists in a tremendously complex balance.

Yet amazingly, all these cells in the body reproduce trillions of times during your life without error and without you having to think about it at all. And the cells multiply in the exact context in which they are required – eye cells continue to be eye cells; liver cells continue to produce liver cells.

If you multiply these numbers by the numbers of people who have lived on the earth over about six million years, along with all the animals and plants that have ever lived, and you consider that all these plants and animals are interconnected in a hugely complex web of life, just the numbers involved are astounding.

When you really think about it, it is inconceivable that all of this complexity at the collective DNA level of all the organisms in the world, let alone all the other complexity in all of the biosphere, came about by chance, from the continual bumping together of a primordial chemical soup on the inanimate earth, from pulverized rock mixed with sea water and sunlight. Yet that is what the materialist paradigm argues.

The materialist argument is that somehow "life," this "extra quality," this epiphenomenon, somehow emerged from a chance combination of inanimate minerals, water and sunlight, and that after life emerged by chance, consciousness was also added as a "froth" to the life force and then self-consciousness somehow emerged, by chance from the supposed froth of consciousness.

It might have been possible in the 19th century, when the body was thought of as something like a billiard ball, solid and "objective," to think of a mechanical evolution. But it is now impossible to imagine how this process could have taken place, now that we know about DNA and sub-atomic particles and the other complexities of theoretical physics. It has become impossible to imagine how chance evolution could have taken rocks and water and, through chance combinations, could have produced such a complex method of manifesting and multiplying life as DNA, where each small unit of life involves trillions of highly accurate, controlled changes, and each of trillions of organisms reproduces over millions of years in an interconnected biosphere.

Information does not arise from nothing, so the complexity of the information encoded in the DNA of just one cell, would suggest that there must be a source of that information other than chance. When you multiply the amount of information in one cell by the untold trillions of interdependent cells on this one planet, it looks like the method of growth involving DNA must have arisen from some kind of comprehensive, universal information source, some form of consciousness, especially when we consider that the DNA of all living things works together as a self-regulating whole, involving unfathomable complexity in its manifestation. That sort of almost omniscient consciousness would usually be called "God."

***

In order to take this a little further, let me tell you about the research of a biologist colleague and friend of mine, Dr. David Scott. David died a few years ago, but he spent much of his professional life doing research on the development of the optic nerve of fruit fly larvae. We used to discuss his research over coffee. I hope I can do his research justice in what I say here.

You may think it is a waste of life to spend so much time on such a seemingly insignificant thing as documenting the stages and nature of the development of the optic nerve of an insignificant creature like the common fruit fly, but the implications of his research are far from insignificant.

David discovered some interesting things about his subject. The fruit fly larvae start out as one cell which has the DNA, discussed above, at its heart. The DNA determines how the cells will divide and what function each cell will have. The first divisions of cells merely add more, seemingly indeterminate cells to the initial one. However, these seemingly identical cells soon begin to differentiate so that one cell will become a head, one a leg and so forth. Yet in the early stages the cells do not have any of the obvious characteristics of those appendages. At this stage, the fruit fly is merely a cluster of cells with little or no definite form.

At some point in the development of the larvae, from the one cell which would become the head, another cell branches out which will be the source of the optic nerve. There will be only one cell to begin with yet, somehow guided by the DNA at its heart, it will divide into two cells with different functions: one to develop into the optic nerve and one to connect with the eye (which has not yet formed). These two cells seem to be floating in the middle of other undifferentiated cells, but they have a powerful force of some sort directing their development.

There is nothing externally striking about either cell, but the DNA is doing some mysterious things. The optic nerve cell continues to divide, producing an additional cell to add to the string of cells which will eventually be the nerve. There is always one cell which is the "leading cell." The leading cell always divides to produce one nerve cell and one leading cell. The nerve is growing toward where the optic centre of the brain will be eventually, although the cells which will develop into the brain have not yet produced a brain. In spite of the absence of a brain, the leading cell of the optic nerve somehow "knows" where the optic centre "will be," and grows in that direction.

David discovered that, if you remove the last three cells on the developing optic nerve, back to an ordinary nerve cell, the cell on the nerve closest to the future brain will change function from being merely a nerve cell and will become a "leading cell," taking on all the characteristics of the destroyed leading cell, even being able to "find its way" to the developing optic centre of the brain. Once the leading cell arrives at the optic centre of the brain, another switch takes place in its function, and it begins to coordinate function with the cells in the developing brain in order to produce connective nerve tissues so that messages can eventually be sent from the eye to the brain.

It must be remembered that, as the cells divided, they were copying all of the billions of steps in the DNA spiral each time they divided. It was as if the DNA was giving the growing cell information about how to grow but, David discovered, there was something more than information coming from within the DNA.

One of the things that he shared with me about his research was that no one knows how the nerve cells "know" which direction to go in, especially considering that the brain they were "seeking out" to connect with, had not even developed. Nor did anyone know how the cells figured out that they had to change function when the other cells were damaged, or how the cells knew it was time to develop connective nerve tissue instead of plain nerve cells and additional leading cells.

The internal information from the DNA didn't seem to be sufficient to explain what was happening, because the nerve "knew" what direction to grow in even before there was any brain to grow toward. It was as if the cells were developing to fill in an already existing energy field pattern before eye, optic nerve and brain had even developed. They were "filling in" the required tissue which would eventually function as part of the whole organism. Since the cause of the "behaviour" of the cells could not be explained from the DNA alone, the facts seemed to demand that the cause be found "outside" the cell, in a "field of conscious direction" which was guiding the development of the cells.

There is a great deal of animosity between traditional materialist scientists and those who believe in "intelligent design" in the development of the universe, largely because many of those who believe in intelligent design are also biblical literalists who believe the earth was created in six days and is no older than 6000 years. David was not in that camp of literalists but he got himself in trouble with some of his colleagues because he found, from his research, that there seemed to be some kind of "intelligent design" in the way the cells functioned. The cells behaved as if, either they had a brain or were being guided by some intelligent force outside themselves. Since they obviously did not have a brain (unless DNA somehow functions on a miniature level as a kind of brain, which is also aware of complex developing organs and tissues) it seems as if all developing organisms, as well as the whole biosphere of which we are part, follow an intelligent "map" of how we should function, before we have even manifested fully as independent organisms.

The only theory that fitted the evidence was a "field theory" which postulated that there are intelligent energy fields which determine how organisms develop. David found that evolution definitely affected the fruit flies after they had grown, and natural selection determined which mutations would survive and which would die, as evolutionary theory postulates, but in the development at the cellular level, another force seemed to be at work.

Many scientists have discovered what David did – that there seems to be a field of consciousness operating in the universe which determines how physical organisms grow or how "collective organisms" like termites and bees or schools of fish or flocks of birds, act. Lynne McTaggart, in her book *The Field*, explores these discoveries and the fate of the scientists who dare to challenge the prevailing "religion of materialism" which says that it is impossible to have such a field because such intelligent fields cannot possibly exist because everything is material substance only. Yet the evidence is mounting daily which suggests that at all levels of life there is some kind of consciousness involved in directing how living organisms develop and interact with each other.

I find it quite exciting, really, that at least some of contemporary science is confirming what mystical writers have known for a long time. Almost all of early science looked at bodies from the outside as if each animal or plant was an "object" just like a rock. In that atmosphere it was easy to think of living organisms as mere "matter." But as scientists look at the inner workings of the cells and the DNA and other forces, it becomes harder to think of the resulting organism as a mere object. Something else is happening which is not accounted for by the materialist model.

The reason I am looking at all these things about cells and DNA and atoms is that, once we change the intellectual model we use to explain life, we can actually begin to use our minds to change our bodies. But as long as we believe that the body is merely matter and energy, we are seemingly hopeless victims of whatever nature wants to throw at us. That is why contemplation is a very important thing to add to your meditative practice, so that you can free yourself from beliefs and ideas which imprison rather than empower.

***

Look at your hand. Examine the lines on the palm, sniff it, touch it, squeeze it and pinch it. It is fairly solid. If you poke a pin into it, it will give quite a resistance to the pin and will hurt.

Obviously, your hand is solid. It is like a mechanical thing when you bend it and it has a solid surface which resists anything entering it. It even has a warning system, the nerves, which make you pull your hand away when something hurts it. But that is only the way it appears to our limited senses.

Now, imagine that you take two of the atoms from that solid hand of yours and magnify them to the size of apples. At the same time, magnify the space between one atom/apple and the next in the same proportion as you magnified the atoms. Surprisingly, the next atom/apple will be about 1500 to 2000 miles (3000-4000 kms.) away! In between is apparently empty space! That solid hand you looked at is mostly empty space; even if our imprecise senses can't see that.

Now, look at the "physical matter" that is there -- in that atom/apple. The atom is made up of more than one hundred sub-atomic particles, each one of them whirling around in its own way. The trouble with the particles, however, is that they are not really particles, and they have so much space between them! Some of them are "wavicles," because they behave like particles sometimes and like waves of energy sometimes. In fact, the "particles" are not physical material at all: they are really intense centres of energy with interesting names like "up and down quarks," "gluons" and "strangelets," besides the usual electrons and protons and neutrons most of us are familiar with.

In this atomic age, we all know the amount of energy which is stored in those atoms. A few atoms can destroy a city.

That solid flesh which is our body is really mostly empty space and a few centres of amazingly concentrated energy. Physicists are now even so doubtful about the nature of matter that they will only say that "matter tends to exist," because it seems to pulse in and out of existence, perhaps into other parallel universes which operate on slightly different wavelengths.

Our bodies really only tend to exist, sometimes, yet they seem to provide a continuity of embodied experience over a lifetime. What is it that provides continuity, then? Is it the body itself or something else?

Answering these questions is important to developing any theory of healing or of the manifesting of the universe. We are not dealing with a chemical machine in medicine or in meditation or in physics: we are dealing with a complex energy system, and we have already seen how this energy system, manifest in the DNA, is also a tremendously complex information storage and information directing system.

The most interesting and challenging thing about this conclusion is that it has been demonstrated in many circumstances that mind and emotions can affect energy in profound ways. For instance, physicists have known for more than one hundred years that if you decide to measure the wave form of sub-atomic "wavicles," they will have energy but no mass, no "substance" to them at all, but if you decide to measure their mass, they will suddenly have no energy wave form but will have mass, even though a moment before they had wave form and no mass. Your decision determines what form they will take.

That raises the question about what consciousness is, what a "decision" is. We are told that everything in the universe is either matter or energy, but I would suggest that there is a third thing which is more powerful than either of those two. Consciousness itself surrounds and interpenetrates all energy and matter. And consciousness, making a decision, changes the nature of the "reality" you are dealing with.

We already know that another "third thing" is involved in matter and energy. Somehow "life" has arisen from what the materialists call "dead matter." Where did the life come from, since it cannot arise from dead matter itself? Consciousness has also arisen and has become an extremely complex self-consciousness – that is, consciousness which is aware of itself and can write about itself as in these words. So we are confronted with matter and energy as part of the universe, but also with life and consciousness as in some ways independent from and able to affect matter and energy. In fact, life and consciousness seem to precede matter and energy and can exist independently of matter and energy.

We human beings are aware of ourselves and of others and have become aware of the world around us to such an extent that we have been able to create tremendously complex social structures, international relations, economic systems, communications technologies and other technologies which could not possibly have arisen just by the chance combinations of chemicals. We have intended these things into existence. Rocks do not produce art, music, literature and philosophy no matter how many years they have to strike against each other in a primordial, lifeless soup.

When you really think about it, the claim of the materialists that all of what we are has come about merely from lifeless matter and energy, with no causative, pre-existing conscious cause, is the height of ignorance and self-imposed blindness. Their claims are impossible to uphold given what science itself has discovered about humanity and the world. That means there are huge areas of ignorance about the causes of the universe which we must begin to explore.

When you consider that consciousness is a form of directed, living energy and that we know it affects the energy which is the matter around and in us, it is not much wonder that we can affect the world with our minds. If we can gain control over our minds and emotions, we can affect the energy around us and within us, intentionally. We can change our bodies with our minds, as I have discovered in putting the body back together after it died and in putting the brain back together after it was badly burned by the encephalitis.

The Prayer of Silence provides some of the groundwork for the sorts of mental and spiritual processes which will begin to open that kind of understanding to us. And the solution is not religion, which has shown itself to be too susceptible to superstition, self-interest and prejudice. The solution lies in opening the deeper spiritual perceptions of the causes of what we call material existence.

That "empty space" between the atoms is not empty, either. It used to be thought that energy was only transferred when one object hit another, like a billiard ball hitting another billiard ball. Now, however, it is known that the energy of one atom is transmitted instantly by this "nothingness" to others around it and even to others separated by great distances. The transmission of information between these subatomic centres of energy seems to take no time at all. It happens instantly.

If you think about it, when you meditate on "nothing," you are meditating on that which seems to unite everything, which makes bridges between everything. "Nothing" is something without which our world or our life could not exist.

It is interesting that a number of traditions refer to God as "No-thing." In the Jewish mystical writings, God, in God's primary Being, is called "Ain Soph" which means "No Thing." That has two meanings: that God cannot be defined in relation to things, which come from God; and that God, as Ain Soph, as No Thing, is the profound basis of all our existence. It would seem that we cannot begin to understand Ain Soph, because we are of the "things," the separated, physical order. However, if both God and the inner "Kingdom of God" are united in consciousness, then we can return to our original awareness of our oneness with God, even if we cannot understand the complexity of God.

Scientists are looking for a Unified Field Theory, a theory of what unites everything in the universe. I would suggest that Nothing unites everything -- and some scientists agree. As we have seen, if you were to remove all energy and matter from a particular space, in the nothing which is left, you would still have something which is very active, something which we have already spoken of, the "Zero Point Field" from which the whole universe seems to emerge constantly. And, as we saw earlier, some scientists suggest that this Zero Point Field is actually "the mind of God."

In Buddhism there is the same sense of seeking "No Thing." It is called Nirvana. Nirvana actually means, "blown out," like a flame. But it is not life which is blown out: it is attachment to the things of the senses and of the world which is blown out so that one can move beyond the "things of the world" to that awareness which is not dependent on those things "where moth and rust destroy and thieves break in and steal," as Yeshua says (Matt 6:20).

Again, we are being led in the Prayer of Silence to a paradox. In one sense the things around us cannot contain God, so we have to let go of things and the definitions and limits of things, to really come to terms with how God, "Nothing," relates to our lives. On the other hand, we are learning that God has manifested everything in the universe and that we can find God in those things, including our bodies. The solution to the paradox lies in realizing what I said earlier, that the universe is not God but that God has manifested the universe. We find God reflected in the things which God has manifested, but we know that God is other than those things.

Therefore, we look for God in the body because, as Yeshua says, the body is the temple of God, but we know that the body is not God. Only our ego thinks the body is God and possessions are God and social position is God, and so runs after those things. We "practise the Presence of God" around and in us, but we do not say that the things around us are God. There is a very important distinction to be made there, and when we solve that puzzle, our consciousness is closer to the consciousness of God.

Look at something as simple as eating, for instance. Our bodies take food and, through an energy/chemical transformation process, change it into bones and teeth and muscles and hair. Carrots become hair by energy transfer. But before the carrots become part of us, carrot seeds take water and nutrients and sunlight and change them into carrots and leaves. Through a long and complex chain of energy transformations, sunlight and manure become hair and teeth.

But research has shown that carrots can be affected in their growth by music, by having people talk to them or sing to them, by having people with healing abilities put their hands near them. Music and speech and attitude and light and bio-energy from hands are all forms of an intelligent energy which affects growth.

Babies, and all people, thrive when they are talked to and when people hug them: they become sick and die when they are left alone. Yeshua's command to visit the sick and the lonely and those in prison has an actual scientific basis, in that our intentional love can affect how others grow and change, and this fact gives new understanding to our role as followers of God's way.

That is tremendous: that means that our bodies are not locked into a mechanical or chemical determinism or prison.

In fact, when you think of it, we are not a "body" at all, in the old mechanical/chemical way of thinking of a body. We are spiritual beings who manifest an aspect of ourselves as complex, cooperative aggregates of extremely concentrated energy which respond to feelings, thoughts and love. This principle is essential to appreciating what happens to us medically when we enter the Silence and begin to make changes to those very feelings, thoughts, attitudes and ideas which hold our energy systems together.

As we get in touch, through meditation, with the calmness and peace of our spiritual nature, our bodies become more at rest as a reflection of that inner, Divine Silence, and many of our illnesses simply disappear because the underlying cause has gone.

Doctors say that many illnesses are "psychosomatic." That means that they are caused by the interaction of the soul (Greek: *psyche*) and the body (Greek: *soma*). They are "soul-caused" diseases. If it is true that most illnesses (up to 80%) and accidents are caused by something wrong with the soul, then what spiritual traditions have said for many years is true: it is the soul which needs to be reformed, remade. A spiritual remedy may be just what we need for our physical ills. That means that if we get in touch with what we are within ourselves, we could cure at least 80% of all our illnesses (perhaps more). And that is where the Prayer of Silence comes in, because I first learned to do meditation in order to cure some medical problems I was having. Only later did I find the spiritual potential.

I know from my own experience that using meditation techniques can help greatly in healing the body. I have been able to get rid of severe chronic pain from a broken back and three back surgeries through meditation techniques. I have also been able to recover from severe memory loss and the complete disintegration of personality following viral encephalitis and its consequent brain damage. I had to learn to put my body back together with Atman/Spirit after the broken back, and then put my brain and thinking functions back together with Atman/Spirit after the encephalitis.

I did not do that all alone, as you know. It has been part of the spiritual training program which Yeshua invited me to take, and in passing that program along to you in this book, I also teach you about healing. Ironically, physical healing is part of the process which led me to discover the reality of Atman/Spirit and the reality of God's Presence. The death of the body made me aware of the Watcher, when I had to use that level of awareness to "put the old machine back together again." The body brings us right back to God – they cannot be separated.

I would like to caution you about an attitude which has arisen in the last few years. People are now saying something to the effect, "You are sick. Ah ha! That must mean there is something wrong with you spiritually. If you can not make yourself better, you are a spiritual failure."

Religion has done enough damage making people feel guilty without the new meditative healing programs doing the same thing. There are many causes of illness which we still do not understand and not all illness responds to the exercises I will teach you. Just because you do not get better does not mean you are a terrible person or a spiritual cripple. It merely means there is a cause deeper than we understand – and the cause may be as simple as germs and viruses. Maybe we have injuries just because we had an accident. Do not make everything into spiritual complication, but if you can learn from your illness and benefit from the learning by becoming a stronger, more positive person in spite of the illness, you have achieved a great deal.

And, of course, we must all die (that is the only way of getting out of this life). There will always be at least one "cause of death" which we cannot heal. I do not wish to create a sense of guilt which says, "Oh my! I am sick. I must be a terrible sinner." That is not the aim, since we all get sick at some time and the causes of illness are very complex -- certainly not a simple punishment for sin.

Our reaction to illness or injury is more important than the fact that we get sick. Meditation, and its consequent change of mind and attitude, can bring about great improvement in our physical health. Looking at life, including our illness, through the eyes of the Watcher, can make us much wiser, more sympathetic and loving people. And when that final illness comes, if we have become accustomed to seeing through the eyes of the Watcher, death will be familiar territory and we will be able to leave the body, knowing that we are not really dead: we have just moved on to another form of being alive.

In the whole, complex array of healing technologies, *the Prayer of Silence* can add another dimension to our understanding of ourselves by giving us direct experience of our bodies from within.

All of this theoretical material has been necessary in order to provide you with the idea of the body on which the Prayer of Silence is built. With that background, we can now go on to do some of the healing exercises which can be very helpful in changing the body with the mind and spirit.

Chapter Nine

Healing the Body with the Mind and Spirit

Over and over, Yeshua told people, "Your faith has made you whole." He basically meant that their attitude to him and to their healing actually caused them to get well. In this chapter we will not work exactly with that kind of faith, but will work with altering the inner dynamics of the mind and body, through the use of the Watcher, to effect healing.

One of the fascinating things about looking through the eyes of the Watcher, and at the same time thinking of our bodies as conscious energy systems, instead of as machines, is that we can learn to direct a powerful stream of consciousness directly into specific parts of our body/energy system. I have outlined below several ways of bringing your consciousness right down to the part of the body which has health problems. Usually one of these methods, or a combination, will work for you.

I will suggest certain visualizations in the exercises, where you picture in your "mind's eye" whatever is being suggested. You may find that you can visualize very easily or that you are one of those who finds visualization difficult, so that you see just a vague image of what you think should be there. It does not matter whether the image in your mind is sharp and clear or not, whether it is in colour or black and white. Just do your best. It is not the quality of the image in the mind that is important – the intent is the main thing.

Visualization is an aid to focusing your consciousness on the part of the body which needs change and it is also a means of activating the powerful healing force in the *theta* level of brain consciousness. Visualization almost automatically activates *theta*, and entering into *theta* makes it possible to identify feelings or ideas stored in the subconscious mind which need to change in order to create healing.

***

Healing exercise one: Visualize light

In all these exercises you should first sit comfortably, close your eyes and enter into the Silence by relaxing, becoming aware of the body, and being aware of the Spirit and the Light around and within you through the Watcher consciousness. Ask for God's guidance. Once you have established yourself in the Watcher consciousness by being able to move your attention around your body, you are ready to do the exercise.

You are already familiar with how to become aware of specific parts of your body by concentrating on them from the Watcher perspective. You also have a sense of how to surround your whole body with light. This exercise builds on the experience you already have and is, in a sense, a concentrated version of your earlier practice.

After you have relaxed your whole body and surrounded yourself with light, concentrate on relaxing further, and being aware of, the part of your body where there is a problem. You will likely find, as you move your awareness to that part of your body, that it appears dark to your inner perception or that it hurts or feels somehow obstructed.

Now, visualize light around and in the dark area. You will likely find that the light won't penetrate very far into the dark area to begin with. You will have to be patient. Continue to focus on the troubled area and on maintaining the light around and in it.

Sometimes it helps if you can move the light back and forth through the dark area as if it is flowing gently through the darkness. It often helps to coordinate the movement of the light with your breathing as well, so that the light moves one way with the in breath and the other way with the out breath. While you do this think gently, "I want this [foot, finger etc] to heal."

Some people may not be able to visualize the light. In that case, just sense your consciousness moving over the area. The light is your consciousness anyway, but the visualization of light seems to amplify the energy from your consciousness. You can actually feel the consciousness flowing like an energy field over the part of your body which needs healing or relaxing. Do this for a while until you feel you have done enough for one session.

You may feel a sense of warmth developing in the area of the body on which you are concentrating. This is partly because the blood flow to the area will increase as the blood vessels are relaxed, but there is also an energy transfer taking place which can be very powerful.

In most cases, one session will not be sufficient. You will have to come back to it on a regular basis over a period of time. Do this exercise two or three times a day for from five to twenty minutes and you will be surprised by the results. Many difficulties in the body will improve and sometimes even vanish with this treatment.

***

Healing exercise two: Visualize repair

There is another method which is more aggressive and which requires a bit more active imagination, but which can be fun, and very effective. It is how I got rid of the chronic back pain I mentioned above. In this method we are consciously affecting a number of systems within our multi-level makeup.

The body is obviously not well or is injured. But, as you enter into the Silence and the Watcher awareness, you move away from the bodily senses and enter into the more subtle realms of your being. At this level you can make use of the hypnagogic imagery I spoke of earlier, that imagery which you usually only see when half way between sleep and waking. As you visualize in that state, you can actually make changes to what I earlier referred to as the "matrix/network body," (the same one which I sensed during the NDE) which are then reflected in the physical body. This network/psychic "double" of the body surrounds and interpenetrates the physical body and is the model on which the physical body is built. Any changes you make in this body, using your spiritual intention, are eventually manifest in the physical body.

By visualizing from the Watcher, you have moved your attention to a level of consciousness "higher" than the physical body, but also higher than that of the matrix body. You are "looking down" from the perspective of the Watcher on the more dense matrix form (what some traditions call the Astral Body) and the even more dense physical form. It also gives us access to the level where the cells are formed or changed and even where the DNA operates. You actually get very close to entering the Zero Point Field from which everything arises. This is where I "saw" everything during the NDE.

This may sound complicated, but when you practice it, you will find these distinctions quite obvious. In fact, when you used your awareness to move light around a part of your visualized body in the last exercise, you were using all these levels of awareness.

In these exercises, you have actually entered into the level of consciousness where you are aware of "spiritual causes" -- into what some traditions call the Causal Body. So, as you change this Causal Body with your spiritual will, you also change the pattern/matrix body (the Astral Body) which in turn affects how the physical body manifests.

Most lasting healing takes place, not on the level of the physical body, but on the higher levels, wherever the difficulty lies. That is why Yeshua often said, "your faith has made you whole," because it is not just the body which is healed, but the inner person (the realm of faith and confidence), which is healed: the body reflects the inner healing. That is also why doctors say that the attitude (the inner being) of the patient determines the recovery. Sometimes healers can heal just the body, but if the inner person is not healed, the illness will return.

That is the theory. Now, let's try the practice.

You may be surprised that this method works at all, but for many people it is the most effective. Here you become a serviceman, seamstress, carpenter, doctor, plumber - whatever suits your fancy. In clinical practice this method has worked wonders on things like cancer and arthritis. I met a man recently at a meditation retreat who was even able to repair blood vessels to his brain using this method, much to the surprise of the doctors and the MRI technician. He imagined he was a plumber putting in new pipes.

After entering the Silence as usual, relaxing and surrounding yourself with light, ask for guidance, enter the Watcher consciousness then focus on the problem area, as you did in the last exercise where you surrounded part of your body with light.

Let's say it is your back which has a lot of pain – I will use my own experience of repairing my back as an example.

As I told you earlier, in 1966 I fell down a 37 foot shaft and broke my back and had two operations to repair a badly shattered vertebra. Unfortunately, I did not know about these methods at the time, so I had to spend seven months in hospital. In 1979 I had another operation to remove a blockage from the spinal cord -- I almost ended up in a wheelchair for the rest of my life, that time, and it left me with chronic and severe pain. The neurosurgeon tried nerve blocks and drugs and was going to implant an electronic stimulator under the skin on both sides of the spinal column to control the pain.

I had tried prayer and relaxation to no avail. Then I learned of this particular method of healing from a number of sources, including research on visualization as an aid to treating cancer in children.

After entering the Silence and asking for guidance, I began to explore the site of the injury with my inner sight. I "saw" that there seemed to be a lengthwise cut along the sheath which surrounds the spinal cord, as well as another cut crossing that one, making an X. This was the first time I had used the method, so was a bit doubtful. However, as is usual when you try this method, a solution suggested itself "out of the blue." It was as if a needle and thread just presented themselves to my inner sight, and I somehow knew I had to draw the edges of the cut spinal sheath back together, especially where the four corners of the X were pulling apart. I began to sew.

To my great surprise, when I stuck the needle into one corner of the X, I got an excruciating pain in my back. That was encouraging! I reasoned that if the visualization caused a pain in my back it must be doing something "real." I stuck the needle into the opposite corner and got the same painful reaction.

By then, I decided this was actually doing something, so I kept going, sewing the flaps back together, closing up the cut. Every time I stuck the imaginary needle into the imaginary sheath around the spinal cord, my back really hurt, but I gritted my teeth and kept going until it was all done. [Actually, you do not usually get this pain reaction. I think I got it just to encourage me to continue.]

Then I just seemed to know that I had to put some healing salve on the wound, so I spread it around (it just appeared in a can, like the ones I knew as a child in India). I then surrounded the whole thing in light for a while (as in the previous exercise) until the sharp pain settled down.

I went back to it three times a day for about a week, repairing any breaks in the thread, putting on more salve, sewing up any sections that came apart, and then surrounding it in light and keeping it in the light and its soothing warmth for a while.

The great news is that I was able to tell the neurosurgeon that I no longer needed the operation to implant the electrodes and have had very little trouble with my back since -- and that is almost thirty years ago. If it gets a bit sore, I move the light back and forth over the area for a while, and it is well again.

Some of the history behind this might be instructive as well.

Because of the pain, before I found out about meditation, I had gone to several healing services, looking for a miracle of healing, and had prayed for a long time and had tried other things. Nothing worked, and I began to think that God didn't care. Maybe God wasn't even there, I thought. Maybe God was just a figment of everyone's imagination. (It is amazing how quickly we can slip back into this kind of doubt even after all the other experiences I had with the NDE. Do not be surprised if you, also, slip in and out of faith. It takes a long time to establish yourself firmly in confidence in the inner way.)

Later, I began to do meditation and realized the potential of meditation to change many of the inner problems of the self. Several years after I had done this exercise and gotten rid of the pain, I asked God, "Abba," in the Silence one day and said, "Why didn't you heal me in one of those faith healing services?"

"Abba" replied in the inner "still small voice" (like the one Elijah heard), "Then you wouldn't have entered this place and gotten to know Me. Wasn't that worth the pain and the search?" And it was! What appeared to be a great evil to me at the time was a way of leading me to a great good. And so I pass it on to you.

But because this is such an important and useful means of dealing with injury or trauma, I will tell you about another of my own experiences to give you a sense of how this works.

A number of years ago I was working in my workshop and caught my finger in an electric planer (it didn't have a guard, by the way, and maybe that was why it was cheap at a garage sale -- later I made a guard so it didn't happen again -- prevention is always better than a cure).

I had cut my left ring finger very badly, with four flaps of finger and nail hanging loose and quite a bit of bleeding. Before I left the workshop, I put the flaps back in place, wrapped some tissue around my finger, applied pressure to stop the bleeding, and went into the house to lie on the bed.

(I must emphasize, if you are hurt very badly, call an ambulance and do all this visualizing in the Emergency Room and later, while recovering.)

I entered the Silence as usual and focused on the hand. I knew that the "treatment" will usually suggest itself from within. This time I had a sense that it would be best to view the hand from a distance, so I allowed it to move away from me down what appeared to be a path. As I examined my hand, very large like a building at the end of the path, the pain was the most obvious general response I got. So, suddenly I found myself holding a large syringe over my shoulder. I stuck it in the wrist of the giant hand and gave it a psychic injection -- the pain actually vanished very quickly.

Bleeding was the next problem. I walked over to the hand in my visualization and there was a door going into the wrist. I went through the door into the hand, climbed up a ladder (which happened to be there) into my finger and began shutting off taps so the blood couldn't flow. Again, after doing this for a few minutes, the bleeding actually stopped.

But those flaps of skin on the outside, which had been cut by the whirling planer, were troublesome. I climbed up another ladder on the outside and nailed them back in place like shingles on a roof. Then I surrounded the whole hand with light for a while as I lay on the bed.

About fifteen minutes after I had cut four large gouges in my left ring finger, I was able to put two small bandage strips on the finger and go out to the workshop to continue what I was working on. I spent the rest of the afternoon out there with no bleeding and no pain.

The finger healed quickly over the next few days. I had to go back in meditation, to check my repairs every once in a while. I put on some ointment a number of times, and surrounded the hand with light for a while whenever I entered the Silence for my regular time there. Now, many years later, I have one U shaped scar and the nail, which was chopped to pieces, is quite normal.

Many people have used this method for controlling cancer (visualizing building walls around tumours to starve them out; or killing tumours which looked like monsters, by stuffing their noses with clay to keep them from breathing); or for arthritis (getting inside and sandpapering the joints and putting on grease); or for nerve damage (visualizing sewing the nerves up again or putting in new electric wires); or even for colds (cleaning all the guck out of the sinuses with a hose and cleaning compound).

If you try this method, be sure to use your sense of humour, because your mind will suggest some quite funny things for you to do at times. I cannot guarantee that everyone will find success in this, because it may be that you have other lessons to learn besides this one, but for many illnesses and injuries it is very effective. The results can be quite startling as you can see from the examples!

But notice what is happening here. We are treating the body, even with severe injury, as if it is an energy system which can be affected by our thought and what we see in the mind's eye. This is not wishful thinking, but an active involvement in our inner being. We no longer think of the body as a machine that cannot be changed. We view the "physical" body as a reflection of a much deeper spiritual process which we can affect by changing the way we "see" it with our deepest inner perception – through the eyes of the Watcher. When we create change in the mind, in the way we "see" our body in the "mind's eye," that change is instantly transmitted to the energy system which underlies the way the body is manifested "physically."

Remember the way the DNA, made up of "only" chemical pairs, seems to "know" what it is supposed to do next when rebuilding an organ, or how the leading cell of the fruit fly optic nerve seems to "know" what to do next when it is damaged, and how there seems to be a "conscious field" in which growth and change take place? Well, it is possible to affect that field with our thought and especially with our visualizations from the perspective of the Watcher, since the Watcher is the basis on which the rest of our thought is built.

The real "WE" is really not a body at all, but something which "makes" the body, which somehow constantly manifests the body from moment to moment and which can change the way the body is manifested in the world when that becomes necessary. Our minds and spirits are very powerful.

This process is not always as quick as is suggested by the examples I have given. I had encephalitis many years ago (in 1991). It has taken all the knowledge of the Inner Way which I had gained through practise before the illness, and all my faith and perception and forgiveness and love and work over the years since 1991 to become, essentially, a new person.

I had to explore past lives and their effect on my present life. I had to rebuild all my relationships and my memories and I had to resolve all the conflicts of many years' standing. I still have some difficulty with certain aspects of memory and can't keep going as long as I would like during the day, because of the residual discomfort in my head from the encephalitis. However, I have moved so far, it is difficult to imagine that, after the illness, I could not copy simple numbers accurately or sign my name or remember people I had known for years. I certainly could not have written this book: I could hardly write a letter.

However, in my case with the encephalitis, my whole life had been destroyed, so I had to rebuild my whole life, not just a finger. It is not much wonder it took so long.

Some things take a lot of time and much work. So, whatever difficulty you have, keep going. Even if it takes years of entering regularly into the Prayer of Silence to deal with the physical problem, you will gradually change in such a way as to bring about healing. Along the way you will learn a great deal more than is involved in healing a broken back or a cut finger. In fact, it may not be physical healing that you need at this point in your life.

Many people fighting terminal illness have found in the Silence with God that they have not been healed in body, but they have been healed emotionally and spiritually before they died and have been able to heal relationships with those they love.

***

The body is usually not the greatest of our problems. More people are afflicted with emotional or mental problems than with problems of the body. And if the estimates we mentioned earlier are true, that at least 80% of physical problems are rooted in emotional stresses and strains, it is obvious that most of our healing must involve emotions, memories, trauma, beliefs, prejudices, or fears.

The exercises that follow in this chapter are designed to help you deal with "problems of the soul." As you go through these exercises, you will begin to get a sense of the general principles involved in them and then you will be able to invent your own ways of finding the healing appropriate to your condition.

It might be helpful to read the rest of this chapter before trying any of the exercises, since the principles I discuss throughout the chapter are important to bear in mind when doing any of the exercises. Some of the ideas at the end of the chapter might help you do the exercises at the beginning more effectively if you read the whole chapter first.

Before we get into any specific exercises, it is important to remember that the daily relaxation every morning will help you deal with the stresses of life and will allow the body to heal itself with no intentional healing involved. Also, the calm and deep breathing will help your body and your emotions to heal because that will bring the added oxygen and life energy which is needed to build and renew your cells. Practicing the Presence of God will give you the reassurance and the inner strength which will bring healing of many of your doubts and fears before you even think about them. Even if you do nothing else, continue the relaxation and the regular breathing and Practicing the Presence, and that will help bring greater wholeness to your emotional and physical life.

Sometimes there are things within us which do not respond to these, because they have deeper causes and something in us actively resists healing. In that case, it is then necessary to uncover them before healing can take place. The following exercises are designed for those conditions.

***

One caution before we go farther: Most people will be able to heal their emotional problems by using the following exercises, but since the causes of emotional problems can be very powerful and painful, in some severe cases of trauma, it may not be sufficient just to read this guide all by yourself and do the exercises all by yourself. *The Prayer of Silence* is very powerful, but sometimes you may need someone with you who has special training in counselling to help you deal with serious trauma or abuse. In that case, *the Prayer of Silence* can be an added aid to your healing but --

It is important to emphasize: if you get into memories which are too difficult for you to handle on your own, seek the help of a professional counsellor.

These people can help you through the memory, and you can then continue with your own growth with greater strength and insight. There is no shame in seeking professional help. In fact, it is a sign of strength that you are willing to seek this help, because it indicates that you really do want to resolve the serious problems with which you may be dealing.

***

Healing exercise three: Changing the body by healing memory

Our bodies are not separate from the rest of what we are. Many of our illnesses are due to unpleasant experiences in the past or inadequate ways of dealing with life in the present. We are only now beginning to become aware as a society of how the trauma of past experiences can affect the rest of our lives, both individually and collectively.

This exercise will help to uncover any painful memories which are causing physical problems.

To do this exercise, enter the Silence in the usual way by relaxing, surrounding yourself with light, asking for God's guidance in preparing yourself to deal with the specific problem you have identified. It is very important to establish yourself in the Watcher consciousness and to ask for God's guidance in this exercise, because you will be activating memories which may make you feel hurt and vulnerable and you need the assurance of God's Presence with you and you also need the objectivity of the Watcher consciousness as you review your memories. Remember, you will be viewing all your memories from the perspective of the peace of the Watcher consciousness, and you can withdraw to that consciousness whenever you feel it is necessary.

Once you have entered into the Watcher, concentrate on the illness or the pain or whatever area of the body needs healing.

As you do this, become aware of whatever memories or ideas or attitudes arise in your mind. Every injury to the body or the emotions will have begun in some event, and is kept alive through the memory of that experience. When you "resolve" the memory, the conflict encoded in the memory usually vanishes, almost miraculously, although the memory still stays with you, but without the stress. The event no longer causes problems because the energy which was stored in the repressed memory is released by being allowed into consciousness.

Just to test if that statement is true, that every body part has a memory, I decided to focus on my left knee because I could not consciously remember any problem there. Immediately, the memory arose of when I was working on my uncle's farm and drove the tine of a manure fork into my knee. The memory is there, even though the pain of the event is no longer there.

If the memory of the knee injury had also involved emotional trauma, and if I had not dealt with the pain of that experience, my knee would likely hurt until I dealt with the emotional content of the memory. We carry the pain in the memory itself. Some memories which arise in the mind when you focus on the painful part of the body, will be directly related to the trauma and some may not seem to be at first. Pay attention to all of them.

Once you have the memory in focus, relive it in as much detail as you can. If it is too painful, just bring a little bit of it into consciousness the first time then let it go and withdraw to the Watcher and its peace. Later you will be able to come back to the memory in more detail, but only allow as much of it to come into your conscious "remembering" as you feel comfortable with, then withdraw to the Watcher focus and allow it to go again. It may take you quite a few times before you can allow the whole memory to come into your mind, if it has been a traumatic one. Do not rush this. However, know that each time you bring the memory into consciousness, you are actually healing a little bit of it.

Also, while you are doing this, become aware of any feelings you have about the memory. Do you feel anger, rage, hurt, guilt, fear, abandonment, loneliness or any other feeling? Explore the feelings. If you feel like crying, then cry. If you feel like swearing, swear. Some people find it helpful to have a pillow to punch if their memory involves anger. That can release many feelings. Allow the emotion to express itself in an appropriate way with the aim of being rid of it finally. (Do not punch a real person, as that will only increase your problems. It is good to be in a private place, because you will feel freer to express what you feel.)

You may find that the tears or anger actually mask something else you had forgotten, and the act of crying will allow that additional memory to surface. There may be many layers of experiences which have been suppressed, which will take time to uncover. Sometimes you will find that the tears have been suppressed for so long you will cry as if the tears will never stop. Allow them to flow, knowing that they will stop. In many spiritual traditions, tears are seen as a spiritual gift, because they are very cleansing and lead to healing.

This process is often painful, especially if the experience you are dealing with has been very traumatic. But by withdrawing to the perspective of the Watcher, you make it easier to deal with the hurt without being overwhelmed. The Watcher is beyond the level of judgment or hurt, and from its perspective you will be able to let go of the problem represented in the memory, because you will realize that you are not the memory or the problem. The problem is something you have stored in your memory from the past, and the event it represents no longer exists.

Once you realize this, you will be able to begin letting it go. That is where your healing begins. But you must do the exercise of entering into the memory in order to find healing. Just knowing this theoretically will not help.

Sometimes you will be able to see the memory as if from a distance. If you can, approach it that way. However, sometimes you will find yourself immersed in the memory as if it is happening all over again and you will re-experience all the original emotions. This can often be even more healing than the objective view, although it is more difficult. It is important to try to keep at least some of your focus in the Watcher, and remember that you are doing this in order to find healing. That way the memory, and the pain you feel, has a purpose – you are doing this in order to heal yourself.

At some point in the reliving of the memory, you will be able to give up your attachment to or your desire to avoid the memory. At that point, you are almost healed. You are getting to the point where you are ready to give up any judgement or blame. It is essential to "know" and claim the experience as your own, in detail, in order to be able to give it up fully: you cannot give away what is not truly yours.

After you have dealt with the memory in this way, you may find you still have another kind of attachment. In order to find complete fulfilment, you will have to forgive the person who was responsible for your hurt and you will have to give up blame. That is perhaps the hardest of Yeshua's injunctions – to forgive your enemies – but he said that because, as long as you carry judgment and condemnation and blame in your heart, you will not be able to give up the experience and you may have to keep the physical ailment which goes along with that blame.

You see, what happened in the past is really just a memory now. There is no person there to blame. That person may have died or have gone on to other things in their life. You keep him/her alive only in the memory. Once you forgive, you let that imaginary person go from your memory. You actually free up a lot of energy – energy you were using to keep the memory and the physical condition alive in you.

If you find the memory that is causing you problems, and then refuse to act on your discovery, you will still be trapped in its errors. If you want revenge, or if you want the other person to suffer before you will let go of the blame, you are really only harming yourself. You MUST forgive and let go of your anger at that point, or you will cause yourself further suffering. When you do allow the memory to be healed, then it is your faith which has healed you.

Here, as elsewhere, honesty, as much as we can muster, is important, even honesty about our own role in the event that has harmed us. Our ego often tries to protect us and to suggest that we had no choice in what happened in the event which caused the hurt. We would like to place the whole blame on others. It is often this which makes us want to blame others, because we do not want to see our own role in the events which harmed us. When we can get beyond blaming others, we will often find self-blame, guilt, anger at ourselves and other powerful emotions hiding in the shadows, attitudes with which we need to deal. You can do that as well, by coming into the Silence regularly and dealing with those additional things that arise. No problem is simple, but the solution is simple – bringing it into focus and letting it go, or asking God to heal it.

It is necessary to be as clear as possible about your own role in your experiences in order to make sure that your understanding of your life experience is not false and deceptive, but is accurate and can lead to the wisdom you seek.

It is also necessary to realize that in some cases you may have developed an undeserved sense of guilt about what has happened to you. This is why clear perception of your experience is necessary, so you can see, not only what the other person has done or what the circumstances have caused, but also know fully your own guilt or lack of it.

Even finding that you somehow contributed to the suffering you had thought was only the responsibility of someone else is liberating, because you will begin to realize that you can now let it go more easily. You will also find you are not trapped in a "victim complex" where you have to keep the victimizer alive in your mind and continue to suffer, so that you can continue to justify your hurt. You can take responsibility for your own actions.

***

Healing exercise four: Dealing with childhood memories

If your hurt comes from when you were a child, there may be a number of errors encoded in the memory. Children often do not understand the dynamics of the situations they are in and adopt their own inadequate understanding, which is then carried over into adulthood, unexamined. It may be necessary to re-interpret what happened by re-living the experience from an adult's perspective. You can do this by visualizing yourself as a child, acting out whatever the memory is. This way you relive the memory from the distance of the Watcher and you see it from the adult's perspective instead of from that of the child. This will give you an adult's view of the events which have been bothering you, and may help you resolve any conflict in the memory.

Another way to deal with childhood problems is even more direct. You visualize yourself as a child, then talk to the child and comfort the child you were. This is very effective in changing your view of the past, since the child you were is very much alive in your consciousness.

When I was a child, I went to a residential school in India, and found that I had to deal as an adult with many feelings of loneliness, abandonment, anger, blame and hurt which came from that experience. In order to resolve the trauma of that time, I visualized myself as a child, playing in front of the dining hall in Ridgewood, the small boys' residence. When I first did this, the child "me" was tracing the pattern in the concrete blocks of the walls, something I realized I used to like to do as a child, but which I had forgotten.

The scene was very vivid. I could sense what the "child me" was feeling, but also what the adult me was feeling. I could then talk to the child in my inner being and actually carry on a conversation. You can even comfort the child and even give the child you a much needed hug. Through a number of these "visits," I was able to help heal much of the pain of that part of my past. It was a bit like doing child counselling with a younger version of myself. But I also learned a great deal about myself as an adult in the process. It was as if the conversation was not just one way, but as if the child was learning something about me, the adult. One wonders if there is actually a communication taking place in this kind of interchange, or if it is just imagination.

I also realized that I had brought over into adulthood quite a bit of blame of my parents for "putting me into boarding." Looking back as an adult, through the perspective of the Watcher, I realized that they did the best they could. I could understand in the Silence why they did what they did, but as a child I could not understand that. I had carried over into adulthood the expectation of most children that adults should be perfect and that the job of parents is to spend all their time looking after the child's needs. This was completely unrealistic, of course, so it helped me to accept my own imperfections when I could accept my parents' imperfections and understand the difficult choices they had to make.

It may seem on the surface that this method of talking to the child could not possibly work, but it is very powerful. It will help you through conflicts which have remained in your being for many years. By reliving the memory, you release the energy which was required to keep it repressed. This blocked energy is often the cause of the pain or illness. I have seen people in their eighties find great relief by resolving memories from their childhood.

A lot of guilt comes from childhood. Children often take on themselves a sense that they are responsible for what happened to their parents or other loved ones. If parents divorce or a parent dies, children often think they are to blame and develop great guilt. If they are abused, they often think that they somehow caused the abuse or that they deserved it, especially if they do not want to blame their parents or other relatives or if the abuser tells the child that he/she was to blame.

Low self-esteem often comes from childhood as well. Because of the distorted view which many children get of traumatic experiences, a lot of people who were abused as children develop a sense of being not only worthless, but someone who deserves punishment. Some adults in this situation will actually look for a partner to punish them and will end up over and over in abusive relationships. They think they are worthless, because they thought as a child that they caused their parent's death or divorce, for instance, so they look for more abuse to justify their belief that they are worthless. Again, talking to yourself as a child in your memory will help to heal these situations.

So, as you go back into memories which involve intense guilt, be aware that some of them may have arisen from a great deal of misinterpreted emotion and a childhood (or later adult) assumption of responsibility which was not yours in the first place.

It is important to try to clarify the whole dynamic of the event you are concentrating on, not just the blame of yourself or the other. It is very often the dynamics of the experience, the pattern or conditions of the experience, which are important and not the question of who is to blame or who is innocent. You will often find patterns of ideas or attitudes or fears which will give you clues to how you can resolve the problems you find.

***

Healing exercise five: dealing with other issues

In all of these exercises, first enter into the Silence, ask for God's help and enter the Watcher by moving your awareness around your body. With this preparation, you can do the visualization more effectively.

If someone else was involved in the hurt, it is possible, as with the child, to visualize the other person and talk to them. You could imagine them sitting in a chair in front of you. It is easier for some people to imagine talking to them over a telephone.

Tell them what you feel about what happened and then allow them to reply. Carry on the conversation until you come to an understanding, realizing that you can always come back to any of these exercises to review in the future. It is surprising the kinds of insights you can get from the answers the person gives you as well as from what you say, so allow yourself to be open to whatever comes up in the conversation.

While going through the process of resolving trauma, it is important to continue your regular meditation, to "Practice the Presence of God," the exercise you did earlier. You will find an increasing strength and comfort which you can get nowhere else. Then, when you enter any traumatic memories, you will be able to call upon that sense of God's Presence and comfort and strength so you can look on the memory without being overcome with emotion. There is always help available if you ask, and many people have found quite surprising strength and comfort in the Presence of God as they confronted the darker side of their experience.

The power of traumatic memories increases as you try to suppress them, because your *psyche*, your soul, wants to be healed, and the only way for that to happen is for your soul to continue forcing the memory into your awareness until you pay attention. When you try to repress negative experiences, you are actually battling with your soul. Once you pay attention and see what is there, then there is no longer that pressure, because you have listened to what your soul is trying to tell you.

You may find, after you resolve something from your memory, that you want to approach the other people who were involved in the remembered incident. In this case, use a great deal of sensitivity for your own sake as well as theirs. You do not want to start a whole new round of conflict, once you have resolved the conflict in yourself.

Ask God for help in this and spend a number of sessions in the Silence, visualizing your meeting with the people concerned, talking to them, understanding their responses and above all, sending them love. After doing that, you may feel it is sufficient to have resolved the conflict in your own mind.

However, if you still want to go on with the meeting with the other person, make sure your contact with them is not designed to gain revenge or to judge or to establish that you were right and they were wrong. Rather, the aim should be to re-establish the understanding, trust and love which was injured. Be aware, however, that the other people involved in your experience will have remembered the incident differently. They may even think you were the one who was responsible for the conflict. Or they may even, like you, have repressed the experience so that they actually do not remember it at all. So, do not require that they agree with your judgement. Rather seek reconciliation and understanding.

In some cases, it might even be necessary just to accept your own healing, and leave the other people to find their own, especially if the other person has died. Once you have done your part, you will have to let the experience go and move on with your own life.

The aim of this cleansing is not to punish others. Rather, the aim is inner healing. If you seek revenge and punishment against the other person, you have merely re-entered the vicious cycle of attack and defence. If, on the other hand, you try to express love, you will be amazed by the results, because you will then have the whole Life of the Universe working toward your healing.

When you are ready to let go of any of the things you uncover, remember the exercise we did early in our practice. There are three steps. First, you must bring the issue into focus as clearly as possible. Next, you must decide to let go of whatever it is, without reserve. Then you tell God that you want to let it go, you ask that it be corrected and you "breath it away," letting it go with each out breath and feeling a refreshing new life entering with each in breath.

That way you know that you have finally resolved the ill effects of the memory and you can go on with your life in a positive and creative way.

***

It is important to emphasize that you should not feel guilt if you are not healed. There are some conditions which, for some reason, do not get better physically. In that case, find peace in the Prayer of Silence and in the things you can do in spite of your limitations.

I have told you of the healing I have experienced -- of a broken back and the effects of encephalitis. The healing from encephalitis took almost twenty years to accomplish, because I had to completely rebuild my brain and its memory banks. As you can see, sometimes you have to persevere!

But I have not told you of the "post-encephalitic" syndrome (much like post-polio syndrome) which I now have, and the constant headaches and considerable fatigue which are part of that. They severely limit the number of hours a day I can work and are very painful at times. I have tried everything to heal those, but for a number of years have been unsuccessful in spite of all I have done. I have learned much as I have entered regularly into the Silence to learn more about my inner nature, but that has not yet translated into healing. Perhaps at some point it will, and perhaps it will not.

But in spite of that, I have written or revised most of this book as well as the first half of *The Thomas Book* while having those symptoms. I have done what I could. And that is what you need to do.

Entering the Prayer of Silence regularly, becoming familiar with the Presence of God and the peace of the meditative state, gives you the strength to continue your life even if you have continuing limitations. You do not have to live with guilt because you are not perfect and you do not have to wait till you are perfect before you begin to live! Continue to do what you can, in spite of your limitations. That way you often discover that your limits are not as great as you thought, and that you can do more than most people think is possible with the limits you have.

***

It took me a while in my own spiritual path to learn the lesson of one aspect of my Near Death Experience. If you remember the story, when I was dying I, as the Watcher, harvested the memories from all of my cells. Memories were not stored only in the brain. When I came back to the body, I had to put the memories back into the cells to get them to function again. It is as if the cells were held together by a web of memories.

What I have been teaching you in the exercises above is an adaptation of that experience. As I advanced in meditation, I discovered that by entering the cells or organs or parts of the body in visualization from the perspective of the Watcher, I could recover the memories that were stored there. And when I dealt with the trauma of different memories, the cells and organs changed as well. The patterns of stress or fear or anger which were blocking the free flow of energy to the different parts of the body changed, and then they could heal themselves.

That is what you are doing in these exercises. You are entering the cells of the body to find the memories which have caused dis-ease, and you are healing those memories in order that the body might become whole.

You will find that the ideas and beliefs and doubts and fears you hold in your mind also affect the body in many ways. We will get into changing those things shortly.

So, whether your problem is illness or injury or addiction or depression or anxiety or any number of other problems, there is a place for you in the Prayer of Silence as you seek for greater wholeness. No problem is excluded from this Prayer, because the Prayer of Silence is a means of bringing your whole life into the Divine Presence.

Chapter Ten

Opening to the Spirit's Intent – Moving from self to Self

"The wind blows where it will,

And you hear its voice but do not know where it comes

from or where it is going:

So is everyone who is born of the Spirit." (John 3:8)

You would think spiritual growth would be easy, since we are developing something inherently beautiful, creative and wonderful. However, spiritual growth is actually hard work, as you have discovered, and the resistance we are struggling with arises from what I call "the material ego," the sense of "I am" which identifies with material things.

This material ego (with a small "e") derives its sense of identity from thinking it is the same as its body, its possessions, its position in society, its professional reputation and anything which has value in a materialist sense. The small "e" ego may also define itself in negative terms – in terms of its poverty or weakness or inadequacy, and may even resist giving up that identity.

The "spiritual Ego" (with capital "E") identifies with God and with positive values like love, peace, joy, compassion, honesty and the like. Strangely, the material ego does not recognize love, joy and peace as worthy goals to be achieved, especially if these get in the way of its social position or its profits or possessions.

In this chapter I use capital and small letters to distinguish the ego and the Ego which are interchangeable with the self and the Self.

Healing the body, stilling the mind and sensing the Divine Presence around and within us are comparatively easy. However, at certain stages of change, as we have seen, growing spiritually is like putting new wine into old wine skins. It can split our old skins, our old way of seeing ourselves, and we do not like to be split! The thing which is split and resists change is the ego: that which wants to grow spiritually is the Ego.

What do we do with the ego, then? Almost every recent book on meditation I have read says we have to get rid of the ego, as if that is what spiritual growth is all about. That may be fine to talk about if you have never gotten rid of the ego but, as with many other things, I disagree because I have done that and know it is not a good idea. I definitely do not want you to get rid of your ego – for a very good reason.

Ego consciousness is simply the way we imagine ourselves to be in relation to the world around and within us. "Ego" is merely our sense of "I am." "I am" consciousness is an essential tool for functioning in the world. It takes many years of trial and error for a child to develop the coherent, effective ego of the adult. There are several medical conditions in which people fail to develop an ego, a sense of the extent and limits of personal space and power, and people who do not develop a coherent sense of "self" have a lot of problems dealing with life.

So, do not even think of getting rid of the ego! That is not what the Prayer of Silence is about.

When I had the encephalitis and lost my memory, I also lost my ego, and it was the most difficult time of my life. I had no sense of who I was. I did not know how to relate to others. It was as if, in losing my ego, I had lost my world and any means I had developed of dealing with the world. I had no protection against the memories of trauma which surfaced from time to time. My emotions shifted rapidly, depending on what was happening around me, because I had no modifying sense of who or what I was. I had no ego, so was like a small child who has no way of relating consistently to the world.

I had to play tricks on myself in order to function from day to day, because I had no coherent sense of self. I used to pretend I was an immigrant who had just come to this country and had to learn again how everything worked, because I didn't even know the customs of going to the store and buying things. I found ways of avoiding conversation because I did not have enough memory to carry on a discussion without revealing I had no idea what I was talking about.

Part of my recovery involved rebuilding an ego in order to function in the world. An important part of rebuilding ego was rebuilding memory of who I had been in the past. Children have to go through this process as well, so I also imagined I had just come into this world as a child and had to build a new life. If children could do this, I reasoned, I could too.

Because of this experience, I would not advise anyone to try to get rid of their ego. Our survival depends on the ego, our "sense of what we are actually like," and we need it. What we do need to achieve, however, is a gradual *change* in the ego's values which will accommodate more of the spiritual things of which we are capable.

One of the valuable lessons of losing my ego was that from then on I knew that everything I chose to add to my new ego, my sense of who I was, was a personal choice which would affect the rest of my life. Most of us who already have an ego are not aware of that. We think that we can do and think whatever we want and it does not necessarily affect us. One of the things the daily review of your actions has likely achieved is that it has emphasized that every action, thought or decision is a choice and it adds to the kind of person you are. You need to be aware of what kind of ego you are growing with every decision, action and thought.

In order to "grow in spirit," we actually need to move from a "lower ego" to a "higher Ego." The lower ego identifies with "the things of this world," with its body image, with its possessions, with its social position and with its reputation. The "higher Ego" identifies with the values of the Kingdom of God – of love, compassion, joy, peace, justice, honesty, and spiritual perception. The change from the lower to the higher Ego cannot be made all at once. As you have been discovering, learning of the values of the Kingdom of God can itself be quite difficult because those values are not at all in tune with self-interest and selfishness.

Changing the ego is not easy because the ego has a lot of investment in keeping things exactly as they are. The lower ego has been working on its self-image since it was a child. It has survived with that sense of self and it is not about to give it up without good reason. It feels it must protect its body, its possessions, its position in society, its ideas and its attitudes because it believes these have allowed it to survive. If it gives these up, it feels it will actually be endangering its very existence.

The lower ego has developed in order to survive in a world it perceives as threatening, so it tries to block any attempts we make to become more "mature" spiritually because the ego sees these attempts not only as criticism of what it has achieved, but as an attack on its very survival. That is why inner growth so often seems to be a struggle. In addition, the lower ego always feels it is fighting for its survival because it knows its world changes and dies. It knows that possessions can be stolen or can be destroyed. It knows that its reputation can be destroyed and it must defend itself against any attack. It is inherently insecure.

The higher Ego, on the other hand, the Atman/Spirit, knows that it can never die and that it does not have to struggle for survival. The Ego does not recognize the threat in the world that the ego feels is there. The ego thinks that the Ego is a threat to its very existence so it does not give up easily.

Our aim is to move from the ego to the Ego, from the self to the Self. If you were not interested in developing the spiritual Ego you would not have read this far in the book, so I can be direct with you. As we move from the ego to the Ego, we often have to find ways of "getting around" the ego in order to let the Ego develop.

In the early stages of the Prayer of Silence, much of what we did was to find ways of "getting around" the ego without letting it know what was happening. Just entering into something as useless (in the ego's terms) as daily silence, was a way of opening up inner perception which could later develop into the Ego. The discussion of the Two Worlds was essentially an exploration of the worlds of both of these egos. Parables are ways of talking to the Ego in ways that the ego does not understand.

Now that you have gotten this far in your spiritual development, you will find it is possible to get in touch with the ego directly in meditation. In the same way as you were able to speak to the child who you were in the past, in the exercise for dealing with traumatic memory, you can also talk to the lower ego because it, like the child's past personality, is a complete personality which in many ways is independent of our Watcher consciousness. There are a number of personalities in us to which we can talk using the Watcher consciousness.

When we enter into the Watcher consciousness, we can talk to the ego about any of its beliefs. It will reply in the inner voice and we can explore its values with it. This is a great way of healing many of "our" limiting beliefs – or our lower ego's limiting beliefs, because we need to gradually shift our identity from the lower ego to the Watcher consciousness which is the foundation of a new, higher Ego.

So we can begin to think of any negative beliefs or ideas as belonging to the ego, and we can see these limiting beliefs as errors we can correct, in the same way as we have been correcting other errors or trauma. When you get far enough on this path of transition, you will find that the new Ego will begin to take over from the old ego, and your personality will change to that of the Ego – to the spiritual values which you are cultivating.

As your Ego becomes more complete, you will also begin to have more confidence in using it instead of the old ego. You will realize that the Ego is not threatening your survival but is actually developing a new way of surviving in the world, using different techniques and values. Instead of confrontation, for instance, you will begin to use discussion and co-operation. Instead of hatred you will use love.

In order to develop the Ego more quickly, now that you are more advanced on the spiritual path, you need to understand some things about the ego. It is a literalist, and can only deal with a literal understanding of its experience.

The ego can band together with others of like mind to form organizations based on the lower ego. We know that "literalist religion" is lower ego religion because, like the ego, which always fears annihilation, this religion bases its ideas and beliefs on fear of annihilation. Beliefs in Hell and in the "end of the world" come from the lower ego. The ego also wants the strict laws, doctrines and definitions of literalist religion; because it only knows how to survive if it is told definite things it can use to define itself.

The religion of the higher Ego, on the other hand, is much harder to define in simple terms, because it is based on inner experience, not on mind definitions. In fact, the Ego will likely not even want to identify with "religion" because it thinks of that as more akin to definition and far away from the inner experience which it thinks of as "spirituality."

The ego always thinks it is logical, even when it talks nonsense. The ego thinks, "I am my body. I am my ideas. I am my possessions. I am my position in life. If anyone, including an aspect of my own consciousness, criticizes my body, ideas, possessions or social status, then they are attacking me and I will defend myself."

The ego is very controlling and uses violence or ridicule as a way of trying to discount any discoveries it cannot argue against logically. Fights, domestic abuse, war, political wrangling, lies, slander or any form of attack and defence arise from the ego feeling it has to be in control. However, because the ego is not terribly clever at defending itself with words and ideas, it often has to resort to violence to strike out at others when it feels attacked.

The ego will use any means it can to defend itself and will escalate its violence as much as it dares, to win its point. When you run into an argument which uses personal ridicule or which threatens any kind of violence, you know you are dealing with an ego which feels threatened. Even reading these words will make some people uneasy or even angry. It is your ego which is responding in this way.

The higher Ego does not need to defend itself or attack because it knows it is immortal and that it cannot be hurt. What we call "faith" is actually the ability to see from the perspective of Atman/Spirit instead of lower ego. From that elevated position we know there is no need to fear or be anxious.

The lower ego will often block certain memories and attitudes from coming to our awareness. This is called repression. We repress memories or beliefs into the "unconscious" because we, the ego, do not want to be conscious of those aspects of ourselves, usually because they say things about us which we do not want to recognize. The ego uses repression as a way to keep itself safe from change, pain or challenge. The conflict you have in trying to bring painful memories into consciousness is actually a struggle between the lower ego, which wants to remain the same, and the higher Ego, which wants to move toward greater wholeness.

Once you resolve repressed conflicts, you are actually helping to strengthen the spiritual Ego. It knows that it can survive better by not repressing material. Honesty is one of the greatest strengths of the Ego, so it wants to bring everything into the open, even if that seems to threaten the ego. That is why Yeshua said that "the truth will make you free."

The lower ego fights because that is the only way it can defend itself. The higher Ego does not need to fight so it can "turn the other cheek," knowing that it cannot be hurt. The way to overcome the lower ego is always to use non-violence so that the lower ego does not feel threatened. Actually, if you are reacting peacefully to any situation, with non-violence, it is a sign that you have brought the higher Ego into play and are acting from that perspective.

That is why it is helpful to withdraw in meditation to the perspective of the Watcher, because the Watcher is the active expression of Atman/Spirit and never feels threatened. The more you do this, the more the new spiritual Ego will form around the freedom and honesty of the Watcher. The exercise I called "Practicing the Presence of God" is partly directed toward strengthening this new Ego in its relationship with God. The more you do that exercise, the more you will feel the strength of the Divine centre of your being emerging into active expression in your everyday life. The confident, relaxed, peaceful, respectful and honest Ego will gradually become who you really are, rather than the fearful, defensive, angry ego you were.

Sometimes we run into blockages where the ego will not let us go any further in a particular spiritual direction. Sometimes we feel like our lives are not flowing and we do not know why. In these situations one of the most effective solutions is to use a form of visualization which is not based on logical, intellectual argument or on conscious control. If we do this, the lower ego has no way of putting up a defence. It does not even know what is happening. Visualization sneaks below the ego's defences. Or to put it in terms of brain function, ego is usually centred in *beta* consciousness while Ego functions mostly in *alpha*, when we do that and *delta*. However, Ego will use *beta* in order to construct logical arguments, but with the intent of *alpha* and lower.

As I pointed out above, the ego is a literalist and does not do very well with symbols and metaphors. Yeshua taught in parables, stories which are metaphorical and symbolic, in order to get around the defences of the ego. Many of his stories dealt with the hypocrisy of the people who thought they were holy. These people thought they were good, but it was a superficial, lower ego, literalist goodness, and Yeshua wanted them to see something more of their spiritual potential. When the Pharisees and Sadducees listened to his stories, their egos felt threatened, but they could not attack him over mere stories, because there were no logical things they could argue against. Almost all of Yeshua's teachings are designed to undercut the superficial logic of the lower ego and are aimed at awakening the higher, Atman/Spirit Ego.

Any organization can be "ego driven." You may belong to one of those, and you may be sensing that it is too restrictive for you, now. Many people find, after meditating for a while, that they must find different people and organizations with which to associate – those which reflect their growing spiritual awareness.

Ego driven organizations have a strict distribution of power and they try to maintain that power at all costs. Whether these are religious, political, cultural or scientific organizations, there is almost always one person (or small group) who is the dictator, who sets policy, controls what is believed and punishes those who stray from the "truth." Members of ego driven organizations (we sometimes call them fundamentalist systems) are not allowed to think for themselves, because the dictators have their own subconscious doubts about their system and know that thought by others will only bring inconsistencies to light. You can usually tell which person or institution or religion is ego driven, because they lash out in violence when they are challenged and they forbid any of their members to question the fundamental tenets of their beliefs.

Much of the violence of our current world is based on ego driven religions or political systems. The alternative, of course, is to learn love and respect, forgiveness and kindness. Strangely, love and respect are all threats to the ego, and there will be a long battle with the self before they can be put into practice universally in the world.

The ego in you will certainly not like reading these paragraphs, in the same way as ego driven religions and political systems in all ages have tried to prevent this kind of knowledge from spreading. When the ego, in its many guises, hears these kinds of arguments, it senses that its time in control is limited, and it will put up a fight. Sometimes it is a vicious fight, because the people who are fighting are really in a battle with themselves. That is why it is said that the battle with the self, with the ego, is the most difficult battle of all.

In order, then, to sidetrack the ego and find answers to problems which are more subtle or more hidden, or to learn of our higher, divine nature, we often have to use a meditative method which opens us to the "Spirit's Intent." As the quote which opens this chapter indicates, the wind of the Spirit blows where it wants to and we do not know where it will take us. We can follow the ways of the world, of the ego, which are predictable, or we can follow the ways of the Spirit which are like the wind, unpredictable. The exercises below open us to the ways of the Spirit and are therefore designed to be as non-restrictive as possible.

There is a whole class of these methods which can be very helpful. I will present a general description of the method, and then suggest some specific examples which will illustrate how you might make specific use of the method. Through this approach, you will begin to get a sense of how you can create your own exercises for specific problems.

Since these exercises draw on spiritual, not just psychological guidance, you can expect that "Spirit," the divine voice within you, will begin to guide you directly. When you get to that stage, you are said to be "Theodidaktos," which is Greek for "taught by God." This is a fulfilment of the hope of Jeremiah, where all people have moved from being controlled by ego to having within them the knowledge of Ego, I AM:

"I will put My law in their minds, and write it on their hearts; and I will be their God, and they shall be My people. No more shall every man teach his neighbour, and every man his brother, saying, 'Know the Lord,' for they all shall know me, from the least of them to the greatest of them, says the Lord." (Jer 31:33-34)

***

Meditation exercise: Opening to the Spirit's Intent

General Method:

In this method you enter the Silence in your usual way. Spend a little time relaxing the body and moving the Watcher attention through the body to deepen your meditative state, then open yourself to God's guidance in one of the following ways (or in another which suggests itself after you have had some experience with these.) It is very important to ask directly, in prayer, for God's guidance, since merely opening yourself to anything that wants to walk into the doors of your spirit is not a good idea – lots of beings would love to find a place to be embodied for a while! Ask for guidance from God or from those who are following the way of God, of the Divine Light and of Divine Love.

In this method we use visualizations of things which are symbolic of opening to something unknown and undefined, something the lower ego has not been able to think about and plan, or something where the lower ego does not have control of what we will see. That way we get around the limited views of the lower ego and allow the Spirit to speak without letting the ego interrupt. Doors, windows, cave openings, tunnels and any kind of entrance can be a symbol of opening to the secrets of the Spirit.

***

Imagine a Door:

This is a method for finding answers to questions of a spiritual nature or for solving a difficulty with which you have been working, and where you have not had success with any other exercises. It does not set up definite limits for what the answer must contain and so opens you to the Spirit's Intent. It does not say that you are looking for a memory or a belief or an attitude. It is completely open to whatever the Spirit's Intent might be for you.

Enter the Silence in the usual way.

In this method, you first of all use "contemplation" and then switch to visualization. Focus first on the question or difficulty you want answered. Bring it into your mind by contemplating on different aspects of the question or difficulty. Explore any opposition you find in yourself to finding a solution, because the opposition will give you clues to what the lower ego thinks about the issue.

When all of this is in focus, imagine yourself standing in front of a door. Briefly ask God to guide you to a solution to your problem on the other side of the door.

Examine the door. What colour is it? How big is it? What is it made of? Does it seem to be going into a building or out of a building or through a wall? What do you feel about the door? Is there fear, anticipation, doubt, hope? Before you go through the door, ask God to guide you as you enter and to provide a solution to the problem on which you have been contemplating.

Now open the door and walk through.

Sometimes you will walk into a room which is familiar to you. One older member of a group I was leading walked into a room in the house where she grew up during the Depression. She had completely forgotten that room consciously, but now she was able to see her mother there, very ill. They were too poor to afford a doctor, so there was nothing they could do for her mother. The emotion of being a girl again, helplessly watching her sick mother, welled up in her and it was good she had our group around to help her through the sorrow of the scene. But then, after the tears, she realized that a great number of things in her life had flowed from the experience in that room. She was able, over a period of time, to explore what was opened to her there and overcome a number of things which had been causing her trouble all her life.

Sometimes the room will not be familiar. In this case observe what you see there. Bring the room into focus as much as possible. What is it like? What furniture is there? What feelings do you have about the room? Is it at all familiar? Is it related to the question to which you are seeking an answer? Sometimes the room will have symbolic elements in it which will have a connection with what you are seeking. If so, try to understand the symbols and what they mean to you.

It is interesting that at times the conscious mind will be blocking things even here. It may be necessary while in this first room (if you do not find an answer to your questions) to find another door. Again, examine the colour and texture of the door, its size and shape. Once it is in focus, ask God for help in finding the answer you are seeking, and then enter through that door. Look again for memories or for symbolic elements or ideas or attitudes.

A man in another group found himself in this situation where he was in a room in his house which did not have any answers. So he went through a second door. This time he was outside his house but not in his yard. Instead, he was in a desolate and dry landscape, not another room. He finally realized this landscape was symbolic. His relationships had become dry and lifeless because he had been spending all his time on his job with no time for his wife and children. With this insight, he was able to go back to his family, re-establish a caring relationship with them and find love and fulfilment there. After that, when he walked again through that second door in meditation, he found himself in a lovely garden with birds and flowers.

Note that the Spirit's Intent in both cases was healing and love, not laws and morality.

***

Imagine a picture on a wall:

In this exercise, after you have entered the Silence as usual and have withdrawn to the Watcher consciousness and have asked for divine guidance, you enter a room, bring it into focus in your mind as above, except, instead of imaging a door to another room, you look around on the walls for a picture.

A picture is more general than a door in its symbolism, so can be of almost anything. Examine the frame of the picture. Examine the picture itself. Is it a photograph or is it done in water colours or oils? What is in the picture? Examine all the elements of the picture. You may find that they change as you examine them. Let them change and do not try to keep them fixed.

You may find that the answer you seek is in the picture itself. It may be of a place you remember or it may have symbolic meanings. If the answer is not there, you can actually go into the picture on the wall and explore what is there.

My own experience with this might be helpful.

At an early point in my practice, I did this exercise to try to see what was blocking my progress at that time. I saw a scene with a large pool of mud in the foreground, then a high fence with the top of a tree visible beyond the fence. It wasn't a memory and I couldn't figure out any symbolic meaning, even after coming back to it a number of times in my time in the Silence over a period of days, so I decided to enter the scene. I immediately found myself in mud up to my neck and had to swim (or struggle) over to the shore by the fence. I climbed the fence, after looking for a way around it. From the top of the fence, I was able to see a landscape of mountains and a beautiful valley beyond.

Once I was on the fence, I realized that this picture was symbolic and also prophetic. The mud told me I had first to do a lot of spiritual housecleaning, like the woman looking for the lost coin in Yeshua's parable; only I was going to be actively struggling through muck. This was a pretty good metaphorical description of what I had to do over the next few weeks in resolving a number of things in my life.

I also realized that I would find barriers (the fence) in my way. I would have to climb over them or resolve them, and that turned out to be true as well.

This was such a productive symbolic picture that I kept coming back to the unfolding elements in it during my time of Silence each day for many months. For instance, once I had cleaned out the things which could be called "mud" in my life and had climbed over some of the fences, I was able to climb down off the fence (more symbolism -- I had to commit myself to the spiritual path instead of sitting on the fence), I started walking along a path toward a bridge over a chasm, with a beautiful valley on the other side. But when I got closer, I saw the bridge was broken and there was a man, dressed like a monk, who pointed to a road that went into a tunnel in the mountain.

I followed the path into the tunnel till I came to a small room chiselled out of the solid rock in the heart of the mountain. There was a rock seat and a small oil lamp. I sat and looked at the chisel marks and meditated there. And that started a long exploration of the meaning at the heart of the mountains of the inner landscape.

It was several months before I had learned enough to come out of the inner mountains of the spirit to find the bridge repaired so I was able to explore the beautiful valley as well. Then I was told I had to leave the valley for a while, since it was not yet time to rest there.

In this case, I came back to the same visualization over and over again, because it became a symbolic journey which I had to follow, applying its message to the development of my life.

Note that this is symbolic but that it is also intensely active. I received symbolic messages from Spirit through a number of people who appeared in the visualization. I was guided in the way my life would develop and then

I had to take the inner messages and translate them into actions in my outer life.

Most of the symbols which arise in these exercises will be very specific to your own experience. They are designed to get around the blockages put up by the lower ego, so will definitely not be advice of a general nature that anyone could interpret. Try to understand how the symbols relate to your specific life situation. You can also expect that the scenes will reveal things about you that even you are not aware of consciously, so it may take concentrated work to understand them. If you put in the required effort, however, you will find rich rewards in spiritual growth.

***

Learning to design your own:

In the above examples you are leaving the "door" open for the Spirit to instruct you in what will bring wholeness and direction in your life, or you are trying to get a "picture" of where you are in your spiritual progress. Notice how the visualizations themselves are related to the words we use to describe what we want to experience.

Because you seek wholeness and healing and love, always ask for God's help as you enter the inner rooms and landscapes. Once you understand the method of opening the inner being to God's guidance through symbols like doors, pictures, windows, bridges, paths or tunnels then you can begin to design your own visualizations.

In order to design your own visualization, you need to do a few things. First you need to spend some time in the Silence trying to understand the inner dynamics of the question with which you are faced and for which you want the guidance of Spirit. Try to discover what its general "shape" is. Use this knowledge as a basis for designing an "inner drama" which will open you to see what you need to see.

You also need to become aware of the kinds of symbols and words to which you respond. They will likely come from your life experience. If you live by the sea, sea and boat images might be appropriate. If you live in the mountains or on the prairies or in the jungle, images from those settings might be most helpful. If you are interested in a particular sport, it may provide you with your inner drama. What team are you playing on or for? What happens if you follow your symbolic golf ball into the forest? What kind of design would you embroider onto a symbolic cloth and where would it take you if you followed it?

Let's take an example. Suppose you have to make a decision between two things. Now that I have some experience in this, a couple of possibilities arise in my mind immediately. The basic structure of the problem is "a decision between two things," so you would seek a symbolic situation which has that double "structure." You might try walking through a door, as in the above exercise, after bringing the matter into focus, expecting to find something on the other side which will help you make the decision, but that is not a specific visualization designed to deal with a choice.

To get more information you could imagine walking on a road (which usually indicates the future). Ahead is a fork in the road -- the decision which needs to be made. You eventually have to choose one road, but in your time of Silence you can actually explore both roads. Walk down each in turn and see where both of the roads lead. This will give you much more information as you explore each alternative, and can help you realize the effects of each decision.

If you live by the sea, you might visualize two boats. See what they both look like. First sail in one of the boats and see what happens. Then sail in the second. See where that takes you. Your symbolic journeys will help you clarify your feelings and ideas and will help you make your decision.

Alternately, you can clarify in your mind the two actions you have to decide on. Are you faced with making a decision between two relationships? In your time in the Silence, ask for God's guidance, then pretend you have acted out the first and follow it through to its conclusion. Then come back and pretend you have acted out the second and follow it through to its conclusion. This will help you become aware of many of the issues involved in the decision which you had not considered before.

You might substitute a cave or a tunnel or some other suggestive opening as a way of exploring your particular concerns.

In order to design your own visualization, you need to be aware of what will open you to the "things of the Spirit" and follow through with that. Remember that you can also enter into the Silence and ask for a visualization which would be appropriate for your particular concerns. Usually, one will be presented to you because Spirit will answer when you ask for guidance.

***

The house of the soul:

Often, the phrases we use can suggest the kinds of visualizations which are appropriate. For instance, we often talk of the body being the "house of the soul." If that is the usual phrase you use, then make it into a visualization exercise.

You can walk though a landscape until you find a house. See what it looks like and what it tells you about yourself. Then explore its rooms to discover some more about your inner nature. This can be the object of many sessions of exploration in your time of Silence, since you will find many things which speak to you of yourself, of your abilities, of the positive things within you as well as of the things which need to be changed. Notice that here the earlier exercises of the door and the picture can be incorporated as well.

Again, these kinds of explorations can continue on and off over several years. Each time you enter the house and make changes in your life, you will find that the house itself changes in some way to indicate your progress.

***

The Path of Life:

We often talk of the "path of life." Paths are often symbolic of the direction our lives are taking, so we can turn that saying into a visualization exercise. Similarly, houses and the rooms in them can be symbols of our whole life: clothing often symbolizes our body or some attitude we hold: cars or vehicles often tell us something about our attitude to our bodies.

You will have private symbols which function for you in a special way as well as cultural symbols. For people from different cultural backgrounds the same symbol may have different meanings. Try to connect the symbol to something personal -- not just something general, since you seek personal enlightenment.

Again an example might help.

After I had the encephalitis in 1991 I was extremely ill. I had lost massive amounts of memory, I could not even copy numbers accurately from one paper to another and even my family felt that I was not the same person I had been. It seemed as if my whole life had fallen apart. But I kept up my meditation practise because, in the years before the illness, I had developed the Watcher aspect of myself to a high degree and knew of its potential for healing. If I was going to heal, I knew it would have to come through meditation and the Watcher.

The brain had been severely damaged by the illness, but I knew that, although the remembering part of me had been wiped clean in many areas, the part that was "really me," the Watcher, was functioning quite well. I used to tell people, "I'm fine, it's just that the rest of me isn't doing very well."

Even though the doctors told me there was nothing they could do, I knew intuitively, from the Watcher perspective, that I could learn what had happened to me and that I could rebuild what had been lost. One doctor told me that most people in my situation became very depressed and entered into despair, but I knew I did not have to despair. I knew there was always an alternative I could work toward.

At one point, I wanted to get a specific sense of what was ahead of me in my future, so I did a meditation with the path image representing my future.

The path on which I found myself in the visualization went through a very uninviting, dark and damp forest. I followed the path, twisting and turning through the trees for quite a long way. Roots and stones tripped my feet and puddles were in the way, so I had to climb around them on the slippery moss. However, I also had a sense that God was with me in spite of the difficulties and that somehow this time in the forest was a time of learning and that I had to keep going.

I kept going from day to day and hour to hour. Life for a long time was like the visualization. I was going through a forest and through slippery paths in my life, but I kept going and I kept entering regularly into the Silence, Practicing the Presence of God and doing the healing exercises I described earlier.

After the initial exercise, which gave me a general picture of my condition and my future, I would check my progress by entering the visualization every once in a while. At first I continued to see the same difficulties, but a bit more light began to appear ahead. Then, after many months of continuing to see the same difficult path, the trees began to thin, the path began to become straighter and smoother and the light shone more brightly through the branches. The inner message from Spirit confirmed that I was healing and it was very encouraging.

I had done a lot of meditation before the encephalitis, so I knew that I was not my material ego -- my body or my brain or my position in society – and

I knew that something else within me was being developed. This was the spiritual Ego.

I knew from the visualization that the difficulties would continue for a while and might even be very severe, so I accepted that and worked within its limits without despair. But I also knew from the visualization that God would be with me the whole way, even when it was very dark, and that I would get through the ordeal. I wondered, at the time, if the writer of Psalm 23 had a similar vision before he wrote those well known words, "Yea though I walk through the valley of the shadow of death, I will fear no evil, for Thou art with me." I felt like I was walking through the valley of the shadow of death, and it was comforting to feel God's Presence with me all the time.

I have come back to this visualization through the intervening years. About ten years after the initial visualization of the dark forest, I found myself still in the forest, but it was less dense now, and with squirrels and birds playing in the branches and sunshine filtering down through the trees. A few months later, in the visualization, I came to the other side the forest and walked down a path which took me to the bottom of a cliff and across a river and into a very interesting landscape. All these settings had symbolic meaning for me at the time, and actually gave me a glimpse into my future.

In all of these visualizations, expect to actually see into the future. Know that messages are sent to you from your spiritual helpers or from God, through this means. This is not just fantasy.

Again, notice that many of these visualizations can be carried over a long period to check your progress. My visualization of the picture with the pool of mud and the fence and mountain cave became a symbolic guide to my progress in my early practice. The meditation with the dark forest, the path and the sense of the Divine Presence was very helpful in a time of difficulty, and I could check it every once in a while as I progressed through different parts of my life.

***

Dealing with symbols

In all of these visualizations you are usually presented with a memory, a scene or a symbol. Sometimes you will not immediately see the connection between the memory or the scene and the question you have asked about your body, your illness, relationships, the issue you want to explore or the general direction of your life. If the meaning is not immediately clear, you need to keep coming back to the experience in your time of Silence and eventually you will see how the experience from the past is related to the present difficulty.

Memories are usually easier to deal with, but if you see a symbol it might be harder to understand. Often the "inner teacher" or spiritual guide presents symbols to us, partly to get around the censorship of the lower ego and also so that we can learn something larger about what we are facing -- not just a specific memory but an attitude or our orientation to life.

Again, an example might help. At one point in my early practice, I was confident that I was getting along very well and was beginning to become proud of what "I" was doing. But then I got into a very dry period in my practice, where I didn't seem to be achieving anything. I would meditate and nothing seemed to happen. I would think that I was very spiritual, but when I meditated I would find that there was nothing within. Sometimes my ego would suggest that this "meditation stuff" was a bunch of nonsense and I should forget about meditating and do something important.

So I asked directly for a message to help me understand what was going wrong. I was presented with a tuning fork with only one side of the fork vibrating.

I knew in my conscious mind that when a tuning fork vibrates, both sides vibrate, so I was puzzled. I knew I was dealing with a symbolic statement but I did not understand. I spent quite a few sessions of entering the Silence in which all I saw before me was that troublesome tuning fork, with only one side vibrating. It was frustrating, because I could not seem to find the answer to the question posed by the symbol and I couldn't seem to get any farther in my spiritual practice. I knew that Spirit had presented me with a puzzle I had to solve if I was going to get any further on the spiritual path.

Then, one day, when I had entered the Silence again, and again saw that frustrating tuning fork and nothing else, I suddenly realized what the problem was.

"I'm not in tune, am I?" I asked.

As soon as I asked that question, the other side of the tuning fork began to vibrate. I realized that in my pride "I" had thought I was doing all the work in this Silence, but I had left out the other side of the tuning fork. Once I realized the it was not just me, my lower ego, doing this spiritual work, but that I had to include God as the other half of everything I was doing, my whole being started to resonate, and I was able to progress further on the path.

***

Listening for the Inner Voice

Another way of dealing with problems is the most direct, but often the most difficult to achieve, and usually comes reliably only after much practice. This method is again to enter the Silence, make sure you are seeing things from the Watcher perspective, so you are not trapped in the narrow world of the ego, ask God for a direct message, and then just sit in the Silence, concentrating on your breathing. Here you wait. In this way you are opening yourself to whatever God sees fit to bring to you but without the structures of the visualizations suggested earlier. It is like the young Samuel in the temple night saying, "Speak Lord, for your servant is listening."

You have already been talking to God in the Silence and perhaps have been getting answers back. If that is the case, this exercise will not be very difficult for you. But if you have not gotten any answers yet, then it will be a bit harder, because you are actually waiting for an answer from God, and our traditions usually tell us that we really can not hear God talking to us.

If someone tells us, "God told me to do such and such," we roll our eyes and think that person is a bit crazy or that their ego is a bit too big. But it is actually possible to hear God's voice speaking to us because, as we have already seen, our inner consciousness, the Atman/Spirit, and God are one, so it is entirely possible to sense what God, the consciousness of the universe in which we have a share, is saying to us.

If you have not heard God speak, it may take some time of waiting to break through the blockages we put up to hearing God's voice. You must be humble to hear God's voice, however. This is not something which is going to make you great, because the expectation of achieving greatness by hearing God speak, is the kind you get from the lower ego, and the lower ego does not hear the divine voice. You wait and listen for the "still, small voice" which is heard in the mind or in the "inner ear." Talk to God, calling God "Abba" if that helps, and wait, listening for the inner voice.

Do not expect that the divine voice is going to tell you all the secrets of the universe, either. Expect reassurance and personal guidance for personal matters, not a great scientific discovery or hidden truth which will make you famous. God does not put on a psychic performance just for your entertainment or self-aggrandisement. Allow the lower ego to melt away, and enter into the Silence and into the Presence of God. Repeat at intervals, "Abba?" "Abba?"

Then listen in patience. And if you do not get a voice in the mind, listen for any other message which is helpful. It may come as a picture in the mind or a memory or a message of some sort. Be open to whatever comes.

It is interesting that children often talk to God and receive a reply, because they do not have the ego conflicts which adults develop. It is good to teach children to talk to God about whatever they want to share with God. They will usually not deceive themselves.

However, adults do need to be a little more careful at times. It is very easy for the ego to suggest things to you and masquerade as God's voice to you. I remember the newspaper story about a group of inexperienced people in an enthusiastic religious group a few years ago who were convinced that God told them to put a baby in the oven to drive the devil out of it: the baby died and they ended up in court, very troubled people.

You need to clear out a lot of the self-deception which pretends to be spiritual evolution before opening yourself in this way, which is why I have left this exercise for later in the book. Always use your common sense in evaluating what you receive, and also examine if the "message" is pandering to the lower ego. If it promises fame or fortune or the punishment of your enemies, realize that it likely comes from the lower ego pretending to be God. Use Yeshua's teachings as a guide to the kinds of things that actually would come from God.

At the present time, many people have convinced themselves that they just need to think positively and God will give them whatever they want – money, cars, houses or a more beautiful wife or handsome husband! They say this is a secret that has been hidden for many centuries. However, this has been known for as long as people have listened to their lower ego and its promises of material things which will enhance the position and comfort of the ego. People are merely letting their lower ego masquerade as the voice of God, and this is a very damaging practice – what in some traditions is called "Black Magic," because it tries to use spiritual power for selfish gain.

You may wonder why I suggest this method at all, if there are dangers in it. First, it is so I can alert you to some of the dangers of the lower ego in meditation. Do not be afraid of talking to God, but be aware of how your ego can lie to you and how you are pre-disposed to believing your ego when it panders to your self-interest.

The most important reason for telling you of this method is that it is an amplification of what I have already taught you about carrying on an informal conversation with God, the consciousness of the universe and the divine centre of your awareness. In the same way that Moses talked to God, "as a man talks to his friend," and Elijah listened for the "still small voice" of God, and Yeshua consulted often with "Abba, Father," one of the major aims of the Prayer of Silence is to make it possible for you to establish the same intimate, informal relationship with "your Father who is in the secret place" in the heart (Matt 6:6).

In times of joy and in times of trial, this relationship will support and sustain you in almost unbelievable ways. And once you have been able to move beyond the self-delusion of the lower ego and have established a relationship with God through the Ego, the Higher Self, you will find that God is never far from you, but is always there to respond to your needs.

As you continue in the Prayer of Silence over the years, you will become aware of how your ego tries to fool you and you will not be deceived. The ego has a vested interest in maintaining things as they are and will not let go of control easily. So you will have to develop what is called discernment. You must practice discernment at all times since, even in advanced stages, it is still easy for us to try to fool ourselves.

You can certainly talk to God about power or money or position or reputation, but be aware that, especially in these areas, there will be a battle going on between the ego and the Divine Inner Voice. That is where we need to keep close watch on ourselves and not act on the instructions of the Inner Voice until we are sure it is actually what it claims to be.

St. Paul wrote of this problem when he said you need to distinguish the character of the guidance you get, and that the "discerning of spirits" is one of the divine gifts (I Cor 12:10).

I do not want to discourage you from doing this exercise, because it can be of tremendous help, but I cannot caution you too much because I know of the dangers of mistaking the voice of your ego and its selfishness for the word which comes from God. If you can talk with God as a child does, with simple, absolute trust, then you will have no problems.

The best method of discernment is to decide if the message panders to your self-interest or if it is self-less. Many people want to use meditation to make money or to give them power over others or to influence the decisions or thoughts of others: that is to be avoided at all costs, because once you start on that road, all other spiritual development stops. Those forces and beings who guide your development will not allow you to proceed further if you try to practice this kind of mind control over others and you will become the victim of your own fancy.

Most cult leaders have entered into this prison of the self and have taken their followers with them. They think their own self-interest and power over their followers is from God. Most of them ask their followers to give up all their money to the leader, to give the leader special sexual favours, often many more partners than the members are allowed, to give up all their thinking and all their decisions to the leader. The cult members believe them and are willing to become mere extensions of the ego of the leader, even committing acts of extreme violence in obedience to the leader.

Do not give authority to others in this Silence, only to God. Test the voices to see if they are from God.

If what you hear is from God, it is self-less. The little self, the ego, the personality which we are so intent on protecting and enriching with power and wealth, continually tries to promote only its interests, not those of others. When we seek God's direction and then pay attention to our self-interest instead, we deceive ourselves very badly, and have to start over to lay a foundation of absolute honesty with God, before we can continue on the inner journey. In that case, we will likely have to go through many times of trial to see if we have really given up the old ego ways before we are allowed to proceed on the spiritual path.

Again, as Yeshua says, and I paraphrase, "Seek first the Kingdom of God and His righteousness, and all other things necessary to your life will be added to you. But if you seek only the things of the ego that is all you will have."

***

Finding Patterns

In any of these exercises, you may discover that what you perceive is part of a pattern of behaviour, of attitude or of belief, and that you need to explore the memories and feelings which are part of the pattern to become aware of what is affecting you.

You may re-enter an experience where you were tremendously angry and think you have gotten rid of the anger, only to find that the anger surfaces again. It may be necessary to re-enter many memories of the same sort of anger to find out why you have that reaction, and then to go back even farther to discover where the pattern began. It may come from a past experience, or it may come from a belief or an idea. Only when you have dealt with it on all levels will you be free of it. You may have to forgive "seventy times seven," as Yeshua says, before you are rid of the problem, so keep going.

The same is true of relationships. I remember one woman telling me she had been in a number of relationships where her partner, husband or boyfriend, was very abusive. She thought of herself as an innocent victim of these men. Then she began to discover that she was drawn into that kind of relationship in spite of herself. She joked that if she was in a room with other people, she was sure to end up with the abuser in the group.

It was only when she realized that she was faced with a pattern of memory and experience that she could do something about it. As she explored the memories, she became aware that as a child she had been taught by her mother that she was no good, that she deserved to be punished, that God was going to punish her in Hell, and that there was no way out. All those years she had been looking for punishment, because she thought she was no good and that she deserved what she got. She also discovered that she actually believed that if she punished herself, God would not punish her. So she sought punishment and abuse because she thought that would "protect" her from God by punishing her now so she wouldn't have to go to Hell in the future.

Once she realized the pattern and the strange distortions her beliefs had caused, she was able to ask God to correct the error of her understanding. She was then free of her bondage and could begin to grow in God's love, instead of being trapped in her mother's belief in God's hatred for her. That discovery literally changed her whole life.

Experiences return again and again because there is something our soul wants us to understand. This is where observing patterns is so important. If you recognize a pattern in your actions or reactions, you know that Atman/Spirit, your "Deep Self," is trying to reach you and has had to use a number of ways to reinforce its message. Once you open yourself to the Winds of the Spirit, the Divine guidance, you can begin to find your way out of your problems and, in the process, develop understanding, compassion and wisdom.

Chapter Eleven

Reincarnation – Dealing with Other Lives

> *When Yeshua came into the region of Caesarea Philippi, He asked His disciples, saying, "Who do men say that I, the Son of Man, am?"*
>
> *So they said, "some say John the Baptist, some Elijah, and others Jeremiah or one of the prophets." (Matt 16:13-14)*

Many people laugh at the mention of past lives, of reincarnation, and even think of it as "un-Christian." However, surveys show that a great number of Christians believe in reincarnation. Wikipedia reports, "Recent surveys by the Barna Group, a Christian research nonprofit organization, have found that a quarter of U.S. Christians, including 10 percent of all born-again Christians, embrace the idea" that we have lived before in some other body and circumstance and will be born again in another body. I am not sure if the clergy in those churches are aware of the large number of their members who differ from the usual beliefs. I know a number of clergy who believe in reincarnation but are cautious about telling their congregations for fear they may upset them unduly.

***

I would like to put in a caution at this point. I have personally found that exploring my own past life memories has been extremely helpful, as I know others have as well. But at the same time, reincarnation is not a doctrine that you must believe in to enter the Silence with God. That is not the purpose at all. If you do not believe in reincarnation, and have had no experiences which point you in that way, or if you are actively opposed to the idea, by all means ignore this section of the book -- but continue with your practice of the Presence of God, with your spiritual growth, and with your devotion to discovering truth as it relates to you. If you want to read this section of the book as merely interesting theory, by all means read it in that light, or omit it entirely if you want. It will not affect your experience in the Silence with God.

***

Because it is non-traditional, I suspect that much of the belief in reincarnation among Christians comes from first-hand experience, either of having remembered past lives or from knowing children or others who have. There are also good reasons, including the idea of justice, which support the belief in reincarnation.

There are many famous (and not so famous) people who have believed in reincarnation because, they say, it makes so much more sense than the idea that we live only one life and then die, being judged eternally on the basis of one life.

The nineteenth century philosopher, Arthur Schopenhauer wrote, "Were an Asiatic to ask me for a definition of Europe, I should be forced to answer him: It is that part of the world which is haunted by the incredible delusion that man was created out of nothing, and that his present birth is his first entrance into life."

It is a haunting delusion, indeed, based on the belief that God creates each soul for the first time in each body, puts that person into social and economic circumstances they did not choose and then judges them on the basis of that one, unchosen life, condemning them to Hell if they were "evil" and to Heaven if they were good. In this belief system, it is claimed that God created the child of the drug addict mother for the first time, put her into a world of poverty where she was raised into a life of prostitution, drug addiction, crime and murder, and then judged her, sending her to Hell for eternity for something she did not want or ask for or choose.

The whole idea is so revolting and unjust that it is easy to see why many people choose to be atheists rather than adopt such a belief. "If God is that unjust," they say, "it is better not to believe in God. If human beings can be more just than that, it is obvious that there is something wrong with the belief in that kind of God."

Interestingly, Yeshua echoed the same argument in the follow-up to his instructions about prayer: "If a son asks for bread from any father among you, will he give him a stone? Or if he asks for a fish, will he give him a serpent instead of a fish? Or if he asks for an egg, will he offer him a scorpion? If you then, being evil, know how to give good gifts to your children, how much more will your heavenly Father give the Holy Spirit to those who ask Him!" (Luke 11:11-13). We can carry that comment further and say, "If we, being human, know how to give good things to our children, would our Heavenly Father be so unjust as to condemn to eternal punishment, those who have not even asked for existence?"

In *The Thomas Book*, Yeshua's teaching about the love of God is firmly linked to reincarnation, in that rebirth gives us sufficient time and sufficient life experience to be able to learn love and correct our errors. It presents a universe where there is justice, where we can be held responsible for our actions and where we have ample opportunity to learn wisdom, by seeing the consequences of our actions, beliefs and ideas over many lifetimes. We are not condemned on the basis of one, short life.

It is quite common for children to relate things which imply they have lived before and have come to this life as yet another of a series. Some of the best research into children and reincarnation was carried out by Ian Stevenson, MD, professor of psychiatry, who investigated cases all over the world where children remembered the names and identities of people they had known in previous lives, even solving murders (where they had been the victims), or finding the family savings which had been buried by "them" in their previous life.

Many people have read Edgar Cayce's works and his conflict, as a conservative Christian, over the messages he got concerning reincarnation. Cayce examined his experiences very thoroughly and finally came to accept that reincarnation was really the only way he could account for many of the things he had experienced. He points out a number of passages in the Bible which seem to refer to the belief.

Yeshua asked his disciples, for instance, "Who do men say that I, the Son of Man, am?" With no hesitation, they replied in a way which indicated that they believed that he was a reincarnation of one of the prophets: "Some say John the Baptist, some Elijah, and others Jeremiah or one of the prophets" (Matt 16:13-14).

In another case, the disciples asked Yeshua about a blind man he had just healed: "Who sinned," they asked, "this man or his parents, that he was born blind?" Of course, he could not have sinned in this life if he was BORN blind, so they obviously thought he had lived a previous life and might have sinned then.

In reply, Yeshua said, "Neither this man nor his parents sinned, but that the works of God should be revealed in him" (John 9:2-3). Yeshua did not say that there was no previous life. His reply indicates that he believed in re-incarnation, only in this case, he said, blindness was not a punishment for sin, but rather so that the healing power of God might be seen working through Yeshua. In addition to the implication that Yeshua and the disciples believed in reincarnation, they also believed in what we call the Law of Karma, or of Cause and Effect, since they accepted that sin in a previous life could have been the cause of blindness in this one.

Many of the early Christians, especially among the Gnostics, believed in reincarnation under different models. Many of the "church fathers" also taught reincarnation. Justin Martyr, Clement of Alexandria and Origen all taught reincarnation or the pre-existence of the soul. In the book of Jeremiah in the Bible there are references to living even before he was in the womb – God did not create a new soul at the moment of birth or conception. Some of the Dead Sea Scrolls, as well as the works of Josephus, a Jewish historian of the first century, speak of a belief in a form of reincarnation among the Essenes or the Pharisees, usually for the virtuous souls who would be rewarded with another life on earth, while the evil souls were punished in the underworld.

The belief in reincarnation also gets into some early hymns of the Christians, who ask that the petitioner may be able to be so virtuous so as not to have to return to another life on earth. In the Book of Revelation, in the New Testament, there is a comment which echoes this hope: "He who overcomes, I will make him a pillar in the temple of My God, and he shall go out no more" (Rev. 3:12). Many people see in this passage a reflection of the belief that, if we can become pure enough, we will not have to return to another life in order to "reap what we have sown" in previous lives.

However, as Elaine Pagels points out in some of her work on early Christianity, it was very difficult to control people who believed in reincarnation, because they could not be made afraid of eternal punishment and therefore did not feel obliged to follow the dictates of the Pope or the priests. In order to frighten people into obedience to the laws of the church, and in order to make sure they donated a good portion of their income to the church, the belief in reincarnation was outlawed and people were forced to believe in the abhorrent doctrine of eternal punishment in Hell. Those who refused to believe were even tortured and burned at the stake.

The selling of Indulgences to pay for the building of St. Peters Basilica in Rome was one of the worst abuses of this fear mongering during the Middle Ages, and led directly to the Reformation under Martin Luther. In "Thesis 50" of his "95 Theses," Luther says that, by selling Indulgences which were sold to allow people to buy their way out of Hell, the Pope "built up [St. Peter's] with the skin, flesh and bones of his sheep."

The church leaders also fought against the idea of reincarnation because they had a competing doctrine – that of the Resurrection of the Body. That doctrine teaches that all believers will be bodily resurrected on the Last Day in the same body they have now, even if it was blown to bits in an explosion. That kind of resurrection of the body is obviously difficult to achieve if people have a number of bodies in different lifetimes.

In the Second Council of Constantinople in 553 A.D., one of a series of "anathemas" was pronounced against the teachings of Origen and the monks who followed him: "If anyone asserts the fabulous preexistence of souls, and shall assert the monstrous restoration which follows from it: let him be anathema." The result was the closure of the monasteries in which this belief was held, and the prohibition against this belief in any form. Interestingly, since the Pope was not at that Council, and since he did not give the anathemas his approval, a number of Roman Catholics have argued that they are not really forbidden from believing in reincarnation, which perhaps accounts for the large numbers of believers in that church.

It is obviously an important belief, and many people have fought against or for it because it does give a lot of freedom to the believer. Also, reincarnation counters one of the main "fear doctrines" of the church – that we are judged by God after only one life and are sent either to Heaven or Hell on the basis of what we do in that one life. For many people, a God who would create souls, unasked, and then condemn billions of them to eternal torment for failing to believe quite arbitrary doctrines, is extremely unjust and irrational.

Reincarnation is actually behind the belief that it is worth meditating and it is worth trying to work toward union with God. Yeshua is quoted as saying, "Therefore you shall be perfect, just as your Father in Heaven is perfect" (Matt 5:48). This text has been the basis for belief in reincarnation among groups such as the Cathars in southern France. It is obviously not possible for most people to be perfect or to find union with "your Father in Heaven" in one lifetime. Reincarnation is the process which gives time for that development, for resolving negative things in life, for dealing with outright crimes and terrible sins against others in the past, and for finding one's way to accepting fully the love of God.

I, for one, have had so many memories of past lives, including the life as Judas Thomas which made it possible for me to write *The Thomas Book* (I write about that extensively in the first half of that book), that it has become part of my being, part of my understanding of the love of God which stretches over thousands of years to draw us back to Union with God.

However, although it is quite obvious that reincarnation is very important in my own life, I do not want to turn this into a doctrine which people must believe in order to practice the Prayer of Silence. *The Prayer of Silence* can bring you to an appreciation of the loving presence of God even if you do not believe in reincarnation. I raise the point here because, while you are doing the exercises above, especially those which ask for God's guidance, you may find a "memory" which is not related to this lifetime at all. You may find yourself in a "memory" of 15th century Spain or as a peasant in China in the early 19th century or an African slave being taken over the Atlantic Ocean in a sailing ship. For many people, this is both troubling and puzzling, especially if they do not know that their memories may refer to some life they, or rather, their Spirit, has lived before.

If you do not believe in reincarnation, there is another way to deal with these memories. You can see them as symbolic, and treating them in this way will help you resolve most of the problems they raise in your meditation. So, finding yourself as a slave owner in the Southern United States in 1802 may or may not mean you were actually a slave owner. It may mean that you are "acting like a slave owner" or that you are thinking of other people as your property and are trying to rule their lives, not giving them freedom.

Also, even if the memory of the past life is valid, it should be seen, not just as a romantic memory which gives you an ego-boost, but as a message of something you need to learn in the present. It has come, after all, not just to fill in history, but because you are looking for information which will help you deal with some difficulty in the present. Your focus in dealing with the memory must always be centred in your present experience and your present circumstance.

If reincarnation is real, as billions of people believe is the case, we remember other lives because there has been something there from which we need to learn. Usually, we will not remember the insignificant things. The only things which seem to carry over into the present life are the important things and, even more often, the troubling or negative things, because it is these from which we have to learn, to correct errors we have made in the past.

So, if you find that the memory you have entered really seems to be a memory and not a symbolic representation of your attitudes or emotional state, what do you do with it? Actually, you can treat it in the same way you would a memory from the present life. You bring it into focus in the present, try to learn as much as is necessary about it and, if you want to overcome the negative attitude, idea or belief which is incorporated in it, you tell God you have finally learned your lesson and want to let it go. I have found it is not always quite that easy, but that is the general process.

If the memory is important enough to have bridged the years, it likely reflects a pattern of behaviour or thought which is still a part of your present personality. I have a number of memories which I have been learning from for over thirty years.

In reincarnation recall, not all is negative. You may find certain skills which carry over from the past. Many child prodigies feel they brought their present extraordinary skill from abilities they cultivated in former lives. I learned how to do a particular kind of sculpting from one of my past incarnations. And you may find that you have something you have to achieve in life which also has been carried over.

In my case, the Near Death Experience uncovered past life connections which then made it possible for me to write The Thomas Book. I had to resolve a number of conflicts with people I lived with in the past and with whom I interacted in this life before I could write that book. And I had to write The Thomas Book as part of a pattern which was planned to span two thousand years.

If you have what you think are past life memories, be aware that they come to you for a reason. Until that reason is fulfilled, you will find them coming up over and over in your time in the Silence because Atman/Spirit seeks wholeness and unity with the Divine in you and others, not discord and separation. The force of Karma, of cause and effect, which has brought the memory to you, also requires that you learn and make changes, and perhaps even make restitution for some of the wrongs "you" committed in the past.

You may not remember any past lives, and that is fine. Perhaps you do not need to at this time. Do not feel you have somehow failed if you do not remember. But, if you are one of the people who does remember past lives, for a variety of reasons, you will find that the emotions and trauma you experience in exploring "past life memories" will be just as powerful as those experienced in exploring your present life memories. The love and the hatred, the hope and the fear and other emotions carry over just as vividly and strongly as from the present. Names and other detailed memories will likely not carry over because that is not usually what we need to resolve. It does not matter if your peasant neighbour was called Jorgen, but if you treated him badly in the past, that is something you will have to resolve. And you can use all the methods suggested above for dealing with past problems.

In exploring many of my own past life memories, I have found myself weeping or sad or angry or full of joy or compassion or love. The emotional content of the memories has not diminished with time or distance. In fact, I have found that many of the deepest feelings of my present life have roots in past lives. And people I have guided through past life emotions have found the same – that the emotional content of reincarnation memory is not muted by the intervening years, and the memories are as powerful as if they happened yesterday.

The traditional Christian teaching about having only one life is valuable in that it makes us concentrate on the present and our responsibility in the present, instead of putting blame on some past event, however far past. We have to take responsibility for who we are now, even if some of the roots of our present personality reach far back in the past. It is never helpful to blame anyone or anything. What we need to do in order to grow spiritually is to become aware of here and now and work from here to develop our future.

I came to the Silence without a belief that I had lived before and found fulfilment in the Practice of the Presence without that belief. Then, through a number of inner experiences, it became unavoidable that I take into account the memory of past lives, at least in my own spiritual path. The memories were just too powerful and too helpful in resolving conflicts in the present and in learning about the soul and the Spirit. I have met a number of people, including devout church members, who have had the same experience -- they have been forced into an acceptance of reincarnation by the experiences they have had.

So, it is not necessary to believe in this, but if you do find yourself in the middle of inner experiences to which God guides you, experiences which suggest that some form of belief in reincarnation is the only explanation, remember you are in the company of many millions of people of all religions.

I do not usually approve of quoting myself, but in this case I think it would be helpful. Following is a passage from the introductory chapters of *The Thomas Book* which clarifies much about how reincarnation works and may help you to understand your own experience if you find reincarnation memories surfacing in your time in the Silence:

Think of the human being, not as a physical body, but as a kind of complex magnetic field. Within this field are a number of frequency levels: what appears to be a physical body (the most dense part of the field); the emotional field; the field of ideas in the mind; the soul field; and the spirit field, which is the centre of the whole thing -- "the True Light that lights everyone coming into the world," as John's Gospel puts it (John 1:9). At the centre of every person is this Divine Light. The darkness of life experience gradually dims the light of the soul in the world and so it is necessary to go through processes of cleansing in order to see the inner Divine Light again.

When you think of reincarnation, think of this total field (minus the body which is replaced in each lifetime) being reincarnated. The emotions, ideas, beliefs and accumulated spiritual perception all adhere to this "entity." Like a magnet, when it is born into the human world, it attracts to itself all the results of its actions and ideas and feelings in the past. Violence in a past life attracts violence in the present life. Love in a past life attracts love in the present life. Each person draws on skills and knowledge acquired in former lives.

Technically, it is not the soul alone which reincarnates. The feelings, beliefs, ideas, attitudes and the results of action also accompany the magnetic field which moves from life to life. Although the body changes, the psycho-spiritual field attached to the soul provides continuity from life to life.

The different fields can be developed to different degrees – the athlete develops the body field, most people have a strong emotional field, some people work on developing the mental field, fewer people are interested in the soul field and at the present, only a very few are aware of the Spirit/Divine field at the centre of their being.

All of these fields can be developed in positive or negative ways. Our beliefs, ideas, attitudes, prejudices and actions all affect the field we are and also affect what we attract to ourselves.

When you remember a past life, you are actually remembering the "beliefs, ideas, attitudes, prejudices and actions," which are closely tied to your present life, because you are the same "magnetic field," only with a different body. All your lives form a network of patterns of action and response, belief and attitude, fear and hope, all of which can potentially lead you to a greater wisdom and understanding than could be achieved with just one life.

***

Meditation Exercise: Working with Past Lives

A final word of caution: My experience has been that we are not given memories of past lives just for fun or to satisfy an idle curiosity. Rather, you need to be actively searching for heightened spiritual perception and growth in order to be given the "privilege" of past life memory. Some people are not ready for this kind of memory, for one reason or another, so are not led in that way. If you do not find any past lives, do not worry about it. There is enough in this one lifetime to keep you very busy with your growing spiritual maturity, without forcing what may not be appropriate for your present stage of growth.

If you are really interested in working with past lives, and if you really feel it would add to your present development, then the following exercise will help you.

The easiest way I know of to experience past lives is an extension of the exercise above in which you went through a landscape and found a building which represented your soul. In that building you can find past lives.

It is good for this exercise to keep a journal, because you will not find the whole of any life right away with one session. Write down what you perceive, read it over fairly often, and continue to enter into the exercise I suggest below. If you do keep a journal, you will begin to discover patterns of experience, belief and relationship which extend between the past life memories and your present relationships and experiences. It is as if you have to awaken to past-life memory gradually. Even then, it is possible that in some cases you may be creating a memory to support some present ego need. It is very difficult to find absolute proof of reincarnation, as many researchers have found, so accept what you receive, and use any perceptions as steps along a very long spiritual path, where you are trying to clarify what is of value and what is not.

In order to find past lives, enter the Silence in the usual way. The Watcher consciousness is very important here because the Watcher is not tied to any one life and can move about in time as it can move about in space. Ask for God's guidance and say that you want to find memories of past lives. Emphasize that you want to do this in order to develop your spiritual perception further. Ask that you may find those past life memories which will be of most help in your present spiritual growth.

Imagine you are walking through a landscape, whatever landscape comes to mind when you start the exercise, noting what you see along the way. At some point in your walk, you will come to a hill. Climb the hill, and on the other side you will see a building which in some way represents your soul. Note what it looks like, what you feel about it. (If you did the previously mentioned exercise, in which you explored the "house of the soul," you can return there and use that as the house to explore or you can look again for a house which is an updated version of the symbolic house of the soul.)

Enter into the building, but this time be aware that you wish to find your way into the basement of the building, the rooms which are under the ground, hidden from the present. Go through the door, down the stairs or tunnel or whatever suggests itself, until you come to a long hallway under the building of your soul.

You will find doors on the right and left along this hall. Ask for guidance in choosing the most appropriate door to begin, and then walk over to that door and examine it. Note what it looks like, how you feel about it, how big it is, and so forth. Once you are ready to enter, open the door and walk in. If you do not feel like entering at this time, because of fear or anxiety, say thank you to God for bringing you this far, and determine to return again another time to explore further.

Remember that past-life recall is often given you to resolve some difficult situation from the past which is manifesting in the present, so this exercise is not to be taken lightly. It will lead you into some real work, and your experience earlier of resolving problems in this life, will be of great help in this process. You can use all your experience of resolving present life situations in resolving issues you find in past life recall.

Once you enter through the door, observe what you see. Don't expect too much at first. Don't judge what you see or try to change it. Just be aware. You may not even know what you are looking at. Explore and note what you see. Spend as much time exploring as you want. Then, when you are ready, come out through the door, close it behind you, and walk back through the hall and out the door into the landscape. Then write down what you have observed.

You can come back to the past life scene again and explore it in more detail. You will also be able to explore other doors coming off the hallway. Each door leads to another life. Gradually, you will be able to build up a larger sense of how your past lives relate to each other and to the present, as well as some of the patterns of belief or experience which have characterized your incarnation experiences. All your lives are connected, and themes and experiences repeat themselves often from one life to another.

Just to give you a little idea of how you might proceed, I will give you an abbreviated account of one of my own memories.

This memory started with a rough, wooden door just to the left as I entered the hallway at the bottom of the stairs leading to the basement. I had the sense that it was a door from long ago, maybe about 1200 A.D. I had mixed feelings about the door before I opened it. There seemed to be many powerful, negative emotions behind that door.

When I opened it, I wasn't quite sure what I was looking at. It looked like I was at the bottom of a dry stone well. There was a steel cage which was obviously lowered by a rope from above. It seemed, as I explored it, that this was a place of retreat, as in a meditation retreat, and that it was associated with a fairly severe monastic order. That was all I got the first time I explored it. I did not understand what I had seen but I returned to my regular consciousness and recorded the experience.

After this one session with the rough door, I was guided to explore other doors and other scenes before I came back to the first one. That way, when I came back to this door, I had a larger context in which to understand this past life.

When I returned the second time, I again found the dry well, but this time "I" was in the cage, only this "I" was in the rough robe of a monk, repeating the rosary. I did not seem to be a very attractive person, either in looks or in personality. I had the sense of being a very harsh person.

I was then pulled up by the rope by someone at the top of the "well" and I found myself in a small, dirty monastery. Over many sessions after that, I was able to fill in parts of a whole lifetime. I did not discover these in chronological order, but as important events to be examined in relation to my present spiritual progress. Almost always, memories of the past were connected to my present experience, so that each entering into the past added something to my present awareness.

That life was a severe religious life but, at the same time I was discovering about that one, I was also being led through other doors into other rooms where I was experiencing other aspects of human life. I was a woman in a number of lives, a rebel in others, a spiritual seeker in yet others. In the same way as we have a variety of experiences in this present life to learn different things, so too we have a variety of lives to learn the many possibilities of life in the flesh.

Briefly, that monk's life went as follows. I shall refer to the monk as "I" because I could feel an identity, however reluctant, with him. As a teenager "I" had condemned my father, a local businessman, because I thought his interest in business and money was evil. I railed against my mother because she was a woman (women were condemned by the church) and she was obviously involved in the sin of sex. I had been persuaded by the priests that sex and money were evil and, in my youthful zeal, had obviously gone too far in my concern with my "salvation," because I was continually condemning my mother and father for what I thought was their life of sin.

Finally, my father threw me, and a servant who agreed with my views, out of the house into the street. I must have been insufferably self-righteous and judgmental. He was not willing to let me treat his wife, my mother, that way anymore. He was angry at what the church had done to his son with its doctrines and attitudes and, although he still loved me, he would no longer allow me to stay and abuse both him and my mother.

I had been taught by the priests and the "Church Fathers," and was very conservative in my beliefs. I had learned the doctrines of that period in history very well. They mostly promoted condemnation, fear and hatred. I even hated my mother and father for bringing me into the world through the sin of sex and birth. I hated women because, in the accepted belief at that time, they were the source of the Fall of Man. Eve had tempted Adam and was obviously in league with the Devil. The only good woman was the "Virgin Mother of God," and our flesh was itself a source of sin and damnation. We had to purge from ourselves all traces of desire or sexuality, all gentleness which would associate us with women. When I became a monk, we used flagellation and deprivation to try to drive the devil of desire out of our bodies.

I blushed in the present to think of the severity of that personality, but I also found that those beliefs actually reflected many of the extreme church beliefs of the time against women, against sex, against money, against the world. It was as if that lifetime had been a concentrated lesson in the kinds of attitudes and beliefs which could lead to the Inquisition and the torture and burning of thousands of innocent women, children and men.

I had joined the monastery and gradually, through my devotion to those beliefs, had become its abbot. It was not a prestigious position, since this was a small institution with dirty, ill-fed monks, practising various forms of self-mutilation in order to try to become pure. It was built like a small stone fortress with a heavy wooden front door and a small back door down a fortified stairway. It had a central courtyard and our cells, chapel and kitchen were off of verandas surrounding the courtyard. The overall sense was of filth, privation, suffering, dampness, cold and condemnation.

I was able to remember quite a number of my beliefs, attitudes and personality. It was not an attractive person I saw there. But interestingly, in the beliefs of this abbot, I recognized in extreme form a number of the ideas and beliefs I had been trying to understand in the present life -- questions of the role of money, sexuality, women, the body, forgiveness, love and other things in the spiritual life. I also recognized some of the source of my present distaste for organized religion and its oppressions. In the present I was actually reacting against who I had been then.

One of the most moving memories of that lifetime, however, was of my father. I had condemned him and he had thrown me out. But our monastery was very poor and we had few benefactors. We would all have starved if it had not been for an anonymous donor. It turned out that my father in that lifetime had given our monastery money out of the love he still felt for his son, in spite of everything. Even as I write this, I still find that action very moving, and it brings tears to my eyes (even every time I revise this text). It is also very much a parable of the love which God has for us, which is often reflected in our own relationships if we are willing to look closely enough.

At the same time that I was remembering that lifetime, I was also led to a lifetime in which I was the victim of the gross inhumanity of the Inquisition – I was a Jewish merchant at the time of the Spanish Inquisition. I was forced to convert to Christianity but still had my possessions confiscated, and was finally tortured and burned at the stake "in order to save my soul." I also experienced other lives in which I felt the effects of this severe, degrading religion from all sides. In consequence, I learned the balance which is arrived at through the experience of many lifetimes, each experiencing a different aspect of the human condition.

I also experienced my death in the monk lifetime. It was a very ironic death, since I died upholding the beliefs of the church of the time against the church. A Papal Legate (supposedly a celibate priest) had come to the area for a visit and wanted to stay at our monastery, but he also wanted his mistress to stay with him. I, as abbot, would not allow this. I told him in no uncertain terms about the evil of sex, of women, of fornication, of the way he was abusing his office, and a few other choice things. This did not go over very well, and over a period of time after that, he arranged to have me accused of heresy and burned at the stake. I even re-experienced the death by burning in the village square.

But all these memories did not all come at once. They emerged as part of a larger process of spiritual discovery and growth. They involved an examination of my present beliefs, attitudes, relationships, fears, prejudices, hatreds and angers. In other words, past life memories from a number of different lives were explored together as part of a fabric of the multi-dimensional being I have discovered myself to be.

If you do follow this direction, you will find you are not just your body or your brain or even just this life. "You," your Higher Self, the Watcher, has experienced many lives and so has a wealth of experience and knowledge from which to draw. You can move beyond the narrow boundaries of the present to attain much greater wisdom as you become aware that you could have been male or female, heterosexual or homosexual, black or white or brown, Christian, Jew, Muslim or Hindu and any number of other things. You will begin to discover in a very intimate way why "There is neither Jew nor Greek, there is neither slave nor free, there is neither male nor female; for you are all one in Christ Jesus" (Gal. 3:28).

If you do decide to follow this exercise, be patient. Integrate it into a larger spiritual practice. Explore past lives some days, practice the Presence most days, resolve difficulties from this life on other days -- make it a part of your larger spiritual exploration. It is important that you do not become obsessed with past lives, but see them in relation to the present. And above all, be sure to ground your memories of the past in your present experience. It is here and now that you are living, and you need to make sure that you bring every discovery back to the present, the now, in order to integrate it into a larger, developing sense of who and what you really are.

***

Regular Exploration of Memories:

As you practice these ways of getting in touch with the trauma or the conflict of the past, you will find that you are gradually freed from the tyranny of the past. Then, when the lessons of the past are learned, you will be able to enter more fully into the life of the present without the fear and hatred and anger and hurt and alienation which has been part of your past experience.

You will also find that, as hatred is resolved, love will rise up of itself within you. As fear is overcome through understanding, you will face life with trust, knowing that everything, even what appeared to be bad things, came from the Divine within you for your instruction. As anger is defused, you will have compassion on the errors and attacks of others. In turning the other cheek, you will be able to help others overcome their sense of being attacked. As alienation is overcome, you will be able to offer help and companionship and healing to others.

Of course, you cannot do all of these exercises all at once. They are for a lifetime of seeking. You can extend these exercises over many years of meditation practise whenever you come upon something in your practise which causes blockages. Gradually, you will grow in spiritual maturity and wisdom.

Get to know yourself. Free yourself of negative influences. Learn compassion and wisdom. Through this extended exploration, you will begin to build an understanding of who you really are. Instead of thinking, "I am the slave of the emotions I feel," you will know that you are someone much greater, someone who does not need to practise anger or hatred or fear to survive. You can begin to see the world with God's eyes which have been hidden within you for too long.

Chapter Twelve

Finding an Inner Spiritual Guide

I leave this subject for this point in the book because I think it is important for you to do a lot of spiritual exploration on your own before depending on a Guide. Actually, though, you have not been working without a Guide. You have been calling on God's help and seeking God's Presence all this time and that is the best basis for all spiritual practice.

The Watcher is the active aspect of Atman/Spirit and, in withdrawing to the Watcher aspect of the self, you are actually entering into the consciousness of the "Higher Self," "the Light that lights every person coming into the world," as John's Gospel puts it. You have been developing an independence of spiritual focus which has given you inner strength and which has strengthened your spiritual perception and spiritual will so that you could achieve healing in all areas of your life.

Calling on the assistance of a Guide or Helper is, in a sense, moving to a more "word based" guidance and it is important to develop a more direct perception of spiritual things before you begin to depend on this mode of help. Even after you do find a Guide to help you, it is good to do a lot of work on your own, so that you continue to develop your own perception. You will not find union with God through a Helper. You find union with God by talking to and becoming one with God.

A Helper can help you to find answers to questions and can suggest ways for you to go, but you have to find your own *gnosis*. There is a saying which is very important here: "Seeking enlightenment is like peeing -- you must do it yourself."

It has been known in all spiritual disciplines that we are not alone in our quest: God is within us and will help us. But often there are other helpers who are assigned to guide us. In the same way that I have been educated to be a teacher in a university, others are educated to teach in all manner of settings, whether in the home or office or hospital or church or factory. We carry on our duties because we have the qualifications and experience to do so.

If we are faithful in carrying out our duties as teacher, learner and helper, we may, like the faithful stewards in Yeshua's parable of the talents, be told that we can take on added responsibility on other levels of being. Some people become helpers after they (that is, their bodies) "die" in this life. And sometimes angelic beings are assigned to be our helpers.

St. Paul speaks of the "great cloud of witnesses" (Heb 10:1) which are ready to help us. He even says of the prophets: "The spirits of the prophets are subject to the prophets" (I Cor 14:32). That is, those people who seek to be in touch with the spiritual realms, as we do, can count on the help of the prophets who preceded them. In my Near Death Experience, described at the beginning of this book, I met three very important prophets – Yeshua, Elijah and Moses -- and have felt their guidance over the years.

In a minute I will suggest a fairly direct way of locating your Helper or Guide. Once located, this Helper can be a very valuable guide to your inner practice. In the Eastern Orthodox churches there has been a very ancient tradition of seeking the inner guide. In that tradition a variety of saints or teachers or even Yeshua are experienced in dreams or during devotions. The Roman Catholic Church teaches that you can contact "Saints" and they can help you. This is valid, as long as you do not restrict your list of helpers to those sanctioned by the church. There are many others from other traditions.

Sometimes Guides appear in symbolic form, rather than in a form we can think of as a particular person. Thus it is recorded that the Holy Spirit was seen by Yeshua as a dove. Most of the Apostles have been associated with different animals through the ages. Moses experienced God as a burning bush. Elijah heard God as a "still, small voice." Ezekiel saw wheels within wheels as he experienced the Divine Presence. In many shamanic traditions animals are the helpers and they bring the qualities associated with them as they guide the shaman.

In the following exercise, we are entering into a very ancient and universal form of spiritual practice, what Carl Jung calls an archetypal experience because it is shared by almost all traditions at a very deep level of the *psyche*, the soul.

The following is an effective way to find your helper. If you do not succeed at first, try again at another time. It may take a number of sessions before you find what you are looking for, so give the Spirit time to work.

***

Meditation Exercise: Finding a Spiritual Helper

Enter into the Silence as usual and ask for God's help and guidance. It is good to spend some time letting go of all the tensions in your mind and body and using the Watcher aspect of the self to feel the Presence of God in the air around you, with the Spirit flowing in and around you. Then pray specifically that in this time in the Silence you may find a Spiritual Helper, if that is appropriate to your present stage of spiritual growth. Say that you would like to be assigned a helper who is at a spiritual level much higher than you so that you can learn more of the spiritual path than you already know.

Now, visualize a stairway. You will walk down the stairway until you come to a place which is totally safe, a place where you are in control. Imagine walking slowly down the stairs, one at a time. Each time you take a step down, you relax a little more. Walk down seven steps, relaxing progressively more with each step. When you reach the bottom you will be in a place which feels totally safe.

A peaceful garden or a warm beach without other people or a cosy room or a forest setting might appear. Allow the setting to be what it will, as long as you feel safe.

I mentioned earlier a young man in a meditation group who had grown up during the civil war in Nigeria. The only safe place he could find in his meditation was a room with four foot thick walls and a steel door, but that was appropriate for him at that point in his spiritual journey. He was able from that setting to progress to one which reflected a greater trust and freedom as he resolved his fears.

Once you are in a setting which is secure, spend some time becoming aware of the setting. This helps you enter more fully into the state of consciousness associated with a place where you feel completely safe and where you are in complete control. You will be able to return to this place any time you want to talk to your Guide, because you will have thoroughly imprinted it on your memory.

When you are ready, tell God that you are ready to meet the Helper or Guide assigned to you. Ask God to send you an appropriate helper. Look around you until you see a person or animal or being on the edge of your safe place. Give them permission to enter and ask them who they are and if they come from God for your good. (What you see may even be a cartoon animal -- in this day of animated movies many people seem to see their Guide in this form.) If the being says that he/she is from God and is your Helper, then you can talk to him/her. If they say they are not, politely ask them to leave and ask another to enter. Finally, even if it takes several sessions, you will find one who says he/she is from God to help you.

Strike up a conversation and get to know this being. Ask why you have been assigned this particular Helper. Discuss anything you want. Usually you will know what you want to ask. Is it related to relationships, to the direction of your spiritual life, some illness or physical disability, money worries or career concerns? You can discuss philosophy or history or anything else that interests you. Ask how you can be more loving, more in tune with the Divine Will. Spend as much time with your Helper as you want, knowing that you can return to this setting again and continue the discussion.

Over the next while, try to follow the advice you get while consulting regularly with this spirit helper. Again, make sure you "discern" the instruction given to you to determine if it comes from your self-interest or if it is actual spiritual guidance. You will usually know, deep within you, whether the instruction is helpful or not. You can ask for God's guidance in this process at any time.

As you get to know the spirit helper, be aware again of the way your own ego and self-interest can intrude into the relationship. Sometimes the advice you get will seem to have something just a little bit wrong with it. You may think, "That does not sound quite right." It is important to keep in mind that the ego will at times try to take over the role of the Helper.

There are also beings who are less than honest who will try to take over from the Helper at times when you are spiritually weak. If you have any doubts, make sure you say a prayer to God asking if the advice is legitimate or not. If you still have doubts about it, leave the Silence for a while. Think about what has happened. When you are rested and when you return to the Silence again, make it your purpose in that session to clarify who is giving you guidance. Observe, become conscious of patterns of advice or experience. Think. Make sure you are not deceiving yourself to try to get away from self knowledge. You might find it helpful to keep a diary of your experiences so you can check on insights and progress here as well.

It is interesting that even Edgar Cayce, who used to go into a trance before allowing his guide to speak through him, went through a phase where there were at least two beings who wanted to talk through him. One was quite a bit more negative than the other, and he had to decide which one to follow.

Often your Guide will be helpful in a direct way or may point out faults that you need to correct or will suggest ways you can improve your life and relationships. Sometimes the Guide will even push you to do something absurd which you have been obsessed with doing for a long time, so that you can see how ridiculous it is and be cured of it. But be observant in this, because not everything has to be done in the physical world: often if is sufficient to imagine you have done the action and then see what the results are in your mind.

If you are afraid of heights and the Guide tells you to jump off a cliff, that is not an invitation to jump off a REAL cliff -- it is enough to jump off a cliff in the mind and feel the hands of God keeping you from injury!

Just a couple of examples of the experience of some other people might help you here.

I must have been terribly proud when I started on this inner way, because when I sought my Guide, he turned out to be a cartoon mouse with a very large nose and a small body. He held his nose in the air, like the typical English cartoon Lord, as if to look down on me with disdain. I said to him, "Surely, you can't be my spirit helper."

He looked at me down his long nose in a proud sort of way and said, "I can leave if you like."

I said no, and immediately learned something about myself: my intellectual pride and its ridiculousness were symbolized for me in that mouse. As I progressed in my spiritual practice, the cartoon mouse gradually changed, so that I realized that not only was he symbolic at the beginning of our relationship, symbolic of what I had to learn in order to move on further, but that the change in form also indicated something of my spiritual development.

Gradually I grew, until my Guide became Yeshua. It was through that relationship I was able to write *The Thomas Book* and enter much more fully into the life of the Spirit.

Another example might be helpful for you as well, since you will see that there are many ways to find the truth in yourself and the one who can guide you. This case also has an odd twist to it.

I was helping a young man who was feeling very depressed. We explored a number of things, including his relationship with a domineering father who wanted him to be perfect. He couldn't live up to what his father wanted, and felt he was a failure in life. So we had a number of sessions where he entered the silence. I guided him as he gradually realized his independence from his father and that he had to take responsibility for his own life and live it according to his own aims.

In the process of one session, he slipped into a memory of being a young knight in medieval Europe. Although they were of the aristocracy, he and his family were quite poor. There were some details in his inner vision which he did not understand and which surprised him, but which were historically very accurate, none the less.

We explored the memory for a while, and then the young man felt drawn to a scene where he, with many hundreds of knights, was involved in a battle. He found the futility of the scene almost unbearable, as knight after knight marched up to the front line, was killed and lay dead on the battle field. Then he was in the front lines and was killed.

He felt himself rise out of his body, and then looked down on the terrible waste, dead men for as far as the eye could see. It was then that he saw an angel who spoke to him.

The young man had almost no religious background, so was quite shocked that this angel, who identified himself as the guide assigned to him, actually was an angel, complete with wings. After commenting to me that it was the oddest thing to see an angel, because he didn't believe in angels, he asked the angel in his mind why he had wings. The angel's answer was revealing: "Because you think angels should have wings." We often see things in Spirit the way we believe they should be.

Well, the deep depression vanished, since it seemed to have arisen both from the disapproval of his father and from the experience of the futility of the battle and the death of so many men. However, the young man continued to have his angel as his guide. A couple of years later he came to see me again. He was frustrated, he said, because his angel would not leave him and seemed to have been assigned to guide him. He wanted to know if there was any way to get rid of an angel, because he didn't want anyone telling him to do more with his life.

I must admit I had to smile at that, and together we had a good laugh. Usually, people want to have an angel around but, in this case, the spiritual guide was apparently given a very difficult assignment by his Boss, and the angel was not appreciated just then.

While I was doing the final edit for this book, I was thinking about this young man. I hadn't seen him for many years and thought it would be good to find out how he was doing. Well, just about three days before sending this to the publisher for final printing, I met him in the grocery store. He went through a period of doing a simple job which did not make too many demands on him, but now he is a manager in an establishment and is also writing a book. He says his angel is still with him, and what happened to him in that short time in the Silence, is the best thing that could have happened to him.

But notice what happened in both these cases, including mine. The Guide is in many ways symbolic as well as being a guide. Pay attention to the symbolism as well as to the help the Guide can give.

The other thing to notice is that the Guide cannot do the work for you. If you are to learn, you must do the work. The Guide, like any teacher, can only put the knowledge before you and then you have to do the learning. All these methods assume that you have to take responsibility for your own development and growth. That is tremendously important. No one else can do your spiritual growing for you.

***

In reviewing all of the methods which open you to the Intent of the Spirit explained above, notice, they are all designed to make you aware of the tremendous spiritual potential within you. They also assume that you can affect the energy system, which appears to be your body, as well as your relationships, in positive, immediate ways by changing things within your *psyche*.

As you continue to enter regularly into the peace and relaxation of the Silence, as you practice the Presence, as you explore each of these methods or a combination of them, you will gradually become aware, from your own experience, of your spiritual potential. You will gain wisdom and understanding and peace and maybe even healing for your body, if that is appropriate for you at this time. You will definitely gain inner healing.

Chapter Thirteen

Mantras

"I am the Alpha and the Omega, the Beginning and the End." (Rev. 1:8)

I said earlier that I would write about mantras, but I left it until this late point in the book for a reason. The kind of meditation I have been taught does not emphasize mantras, those repeated words or sounds which are the centre of some traditions. Here I will explain the reasons for this alternate emphasis and also about mantras themselves and how you can use them as part of your meditative practice if you want to.

As you become more advanced in your practice, you may want to experiment with a number of different meditation exercises you hear or read about. Be open to other possibilities. This book does not in any way exhaust the possible benefits to be found in other forms of meditation, nor does it forbid the use of other methods. But before you try any other methods, enter the Silence as usual and ask God to guide you, so that what you do is consistent with the values you have been developing in your relationship with the "God within."

A mantra is a sound or a phrase which is repeated over and over during meditation. It is usually co-ordinated with the breathing. It can be said out loud or can be an interior sound. Saying the mantra in the interior, silent way is more effective, but at the beginning, and in groups, the mantra is usually chanted out loud. Gregorian chants, sung by many voices, are a form of mantra, as are many of the repetitive songs sung in churches.

The Russian Orthodox Church has a tradition in which a repeated mantra, usually the "Jesus Prayer," which we will discuss shortly, moves from the spoken form (thousands of times a day) to the non-verbal form and then, at some point, becomes the "Prayer of the Heart," where the whole of life becomes suffused with prayer.

Some mantras are even whole poems, like selected Psalms or passages of Scripture or prayers like the Lord's Prayer. The Roman Catholic Church has a number of prayers which are repeated and counted on the rosary – like the "Our Father," "Hail Mary" and others. Many traditions, including the Hindu and Buddhist traditions, use a rosary to keep track of the number of times a prayer or mantra is said.

Mantras vary a great deal from tradition to tradition. In some traditions, mantras are one word specially designed for each student by the guru, and are kept secret, while others are said by everyone and are common to the whole community. In the Buddhist, Muslim and Hindu traditions, long passages from the scriptures are recited from memory as mantras.

Obviously, we cannot consider everything about mantras here. However, I would like to take up two aspects of mantras which are important for you to consider if you decide to take this path. Again, I emphasize that they are not essential to your progress. You can achieve Divine Union without using mantras, but they are helpful at some time for some people on their journey, as part of a larger program, and you might want to try them to see if they are suitable for you.

The meditation I have introduced you to here might be called an "awareness meditation." In this meditation you are asked to become aware in the Silence of as many aspects of your complex nature as possible. You are trying to bring everything about you into the Silence, in order that it be transformed by that direct and conscious contact with God. You have gotten to know your body and its connection to the events of the day, to emotions, the ego, memories, beliefs, relationships, ideas, attitudes, past lives and more. You have become aware of the tremendous potential of the Watcher to transform your life. You have also become aware of the Divine Presence around and within you.

There is almost always a centre of focus in meditation, and the mantra is the centre of focus for many traditions. Concentrating on the breath or on a candle flame or on music can provide the required focus.

In the Prayer of Silence, we have been seeing from the perspective of the Watcher, but the body has provided the unifying focus. From the body, we connect to everything else, and see everything in our lives as it is reflected in the body. The body even reveals how God is manifest in us.

The teaching I have received has guided me away from mantras for most of my time in this training program, because in many traditions the mantra is used, not for awareness, but to repress awareness. Repeating the mantra helps bring concentration by activating the speech centres of the brain and, once the speech centre is activated, it is difficult to be aware of anything else. The way the mantra works is by suppressing other thoughts and sounds. Try to say, "crocodile," over and over and at the same time try to think any other words or phrases. The repeated word blocks access to other words or ideas. For this purpose, almost any word will do, including "crocodile."

The theory behind this is that, in blocking the "wandering thoughts" we spoke of earlier, the mind is gradually forced to perceive higher realities, to switch into trance-like states which transcend ordinary consciousness. And that is fine to an extent, but I have met some advanced meditators who seem to be very unaware of their everyday reality and the effect of emotion and relationship on their spiritual nature. They can "transcend" everyday reality in meditation, but have a great deal of difficulty dealing with the world around and in them. Mantra meditation tends to emphasize withdrawal from awareness, rather than involvement in awareness.

The "awareness meditation" you have been practising here, is designed to make you familiar with all the aspects of your life which you have to deal with everyday, as well as with your spiritual nature. Suppression is prevented here, not encouraged, and your meditation exercises actually make it impossible for you to avoid the ideas and feelings which arise within you. In this kind of meditation, you develop transcendental states, the Samadhi or Satori which other traditions achieve, but you also deal with the conflicts which are part of your inner nature and which must be resolved and integrated before you can become whole.

Once you have begun to develop a sense of integration in your inner being, then it can be valuable at times to employ mantras to give an added focus and to take you into other kinds of spiritual awareness. In my discussion of mantras here, then, I will be emphasizing other forms of awareness, in line with what you have been doing already, and will not suggest that you use mantras to suppress any kind of inner awareness. In fact, if you find any emotional conflicts arising in you while doing mantra meditation, you should stop that meditation, resolve the conflict using methods you have already learned, and then resume your mantra meditation.

That is why I leave a discussion of mantras to this point in the book, so that you have the knowledge and experience to be able to move into higher states of consciousness without the burden of unresolved personal issues.

The two aspects of mantras I will discuss here are sound and meaning, along with their effects. I will not assign mantras to you, since that is not my tradition. But if you wish to choose a mantra, what follows will give you sufficient information to make an informed choice.

***

The sound of the mantra

A repeated mantra should not be harsh or jarring on the inner being. It should have a sonorous quality which reverberates in the main parts of the body. In fact, the sounds of mantras are often associated with energy centres in the body. The lower sounds usually resonate near the base of the spine, while the higher sounds move toward the head. Often, the first part of the mantra is chanted while concentrating on the base of the spine and the sound gradually flows, with the concentration, up the back and into the head. In the Eastern tradition, there are even separate mantras, called "bija" or seed mantras, for concentrating on the different energy centres, called "chakras" (pronounced with a hard "chack-raa" in Sanskrit, not the popular Western "shaaa-kraa").

There is a Tibetan Buddhist chant which actually vibrates in chords, so that you are resonating at the base of the spine, several points higher (usually the heart or throat) and in the head, all at the same time. Once learned, this can be an amazingly unifying experience, since it brings a number of energy centres into harmony. Practicing it regularly has a blissful quality to it.

A few years ago, our family was travelling in India, and we went to the Elora Caves near Mumbai (Bombay). These cave temples were carved out of the solid rock about two thousand years ago by Buddhist and Hindu monks. One of these temples had a very high, corrugated stone ceiling, as well as several of the main Buddhist symbols, so it was obviously a place of Buddhist meditation. We were wondering why it was shaped as it was. Thinking it was likely designed for chanted meditation, we started chanting the almost universal mantra, "OM," over and over, to see what effect it would have in that space. It reverberated back and forth through the sanctuary, and the ribbed ceiling made it echo more and more, building up the volume and the depth of the chant. It sounded a bit like the "Music of the Spheres" I will discuss later in this chapter. A young couple near the back of the temple started playing flutes as we chanted, and the effect was amazingly beautiful. It was obvious that the temple had been designed for its acoustics, to be a place for chanting mantras.

You will find that most mantras which rely on sound have a lot of M's and N's in them, like the OM which is used widely in the East, since these consonants resonate in the chest, or heart chakra, and head, or higher chakras. The vowels are usually long vowels, since part of the resonance involves the alternating consonants and long vowels. Thus we have meditation words, or mantras from the Christian tradition like "Maranatha" or "Amen." When chanted or sung, the vowels are usually lengthened, the "a's" are made into long "a's," the "o's" into long "o's" and so forth, each syllable distinct. Many people find singing the "Amen" very moving, and part of the effect likely arises from it having some of the standard sounds of the "OM" mantra.

In choosing a mantra, you must make sure it does not destroy some other meaning which the word has for you. For instance, Yeshua called God "Abba," the Aramaic word for "Dad." This word expresses the absolute trust and closeness which a child has with a parent. One scholar has even said that the only really original teaching of Yeshua is his use of "Abba" for God. It is a name you have already used while "Practicing the Presence." When you use it in your conversations with God, it can be very moving.

If you use "Abba" as a repeated mantra, repeating it over and over, it will lose the sense of relationship. That is why I recommend you not use a word for a mantra, which has an important meaning in another context.

However, there is another word which Yeshua taught his disciples, which has the qualities of a mantra. In the "Our Father which art in Heaven" prayer, the Aramaic language he used, refers to "Our Father" as "Abwoon," likely pronounced "Ab-(w)-oon," with the "w" almost silent. If you chant that name, you will find it resonates both in sound and meaning.

***

Meditation exercise: chanting a mantra

In order to chant this, or any other mantra, first enter the Silence by the usual means of asking for God's guidance, relaxing, becoming aware of the Watcher and of the body and letting go of tensions. To chant Abwoon, coordinate the word, your breath and the way your attention moves through the body.

As you breathe in, visualize the "Aaaab" resonating and moving from the base of the spine up to the top of the head. As you breathe out, visualize the "woooon" moving from the top of the head, down the front of your body, to the base of the spine. (An alternate movement is from the heels to the top of the head, then from the top of the head to the feet, so your whole body is enveloped in the chant.) Because you know how to see from the Watcher, this meditation will be even more effective than if you did not know about that aspect of your consciousness, because you are now causing the sound and the meaning to resonate at fundamental levels of your being.

Be aware of the sound and the meaning, since they are both important. Abwoon is the word for father at the beginning of the Lord's Prayer in Aramaic, but is also the word for the source of life, and in Aramaic the distinction between father and mother disappears in this word and it is more like saying, "father/mother." It is also related to the process of manifestation and birth, almost like "womb." As you chant, sense the vibration of the word. Let the "(w)oon" resonate in the head and down through the body, as if the skull and the chest are the roof of the temple.

At first, chant out loud. As you become aware of the way the mantra works in the body, you can chant silently, concentrating in an interior way. Explore the differences in the vocalized chant and the silent repetition of the mantra.

It does not take long for this kind of chant to move your consciousness into an altered state. Ask for God's guidance and then let your consciousness go where it wishes.

If using mantras in a group, you can chant two ways. Usually the chant is in unison, with someone leading, especially if it is a longer mantra. This keeps everyone on track. But with a shorter, one or two syllable mantra, the chant can also involve each person developing their own pace, so that the sounds overlap. While chanting, let yourself relax into the sound.

Usually, two weeks of regular chanting is needed to sense a difference in the way your system reacts to itself and the world because of the mantra. However, now that you have been doing the kind of transformative meditation learned in the Prayer of Silence, and since you know about the powerful effects of the Watcher, you will find that the mantra can lead you very quickly to an altered, spiritual state because you do not have to worry about all the distractions which you have already resolved.

You may find that the word "womb" has meaning for you as a chanted mantra. In this case, the sound is appropriate and the meaning can be seen as not just the place where a foetus is carried, but extended into the sense of the Divine source of life, the Divine Feminine, the whole miracle of growth and birth, almost like Abwoon, where the distinction of male and female in the Divine disappears into a dynamic unity. Sense how the meaning and the sound relate to the pulsing of life and the universe around you and feel yourself as part of the creative miracle.

All of these mantra sounds are related to an ancient mantra which is used extensively in Hinduism and Buddhism but which pre-dates those religions, going back into the mists of time. It is the "OM" which we chanted in the cave in Elora. But it is not just something from Hinduism and Buddhism. I was surprised to discover that it has an interesting relation to Christianity as well.

Christianity grew up in the Middle East, at a time when many traditions were influencing each other. One of the most ancient of these traditions spread from India, passing through trade routes, routes of conquest, cultural influence and language transfer. The ancient Hebrew, Greek and Egyptian languages have words which are derived from ancient Sanskrit, the language of the Hindu scriptures and theology. Since theological language spread from India to Hebrew, Greek and the Egyptian languages, it is fair to assume that the ideas themselves also came with them.

Buddhist missionaries were active in the Middle East during the first centuries of the present era, even getting as far west as England. Buddhism, Judaism and Christianity influenced each other at that time. Some researchers think that the Essenes, a Jewish sect at the time of Yeshua, believed in a form of "Jewish Buddhism" -- and much evidence suggests that Yeshua was also a member of the Essene community.

Some traditions also claim that Yeshua went to India to learn: after all, that is where tradition also says at least one of the Wise Men came from who brought their gifts to the young Yeshua (actually from Ujjain, the city where I spent part of my childhood.)

The ancient traditions say that the universe began with a sound, a vibration, and that creation continues through vibration. The Bible says that God created by sound in saying, "Let there be." John's gospel says, "In the beginning was the Word." Even scientists say that the universe arises from a vibration.

The Universal Sound has come into the writings of many traditions and we can begin to trace it in sounds like the "oon" or "uum" or "aum" of words like "abwoon," "womb," "amen," or "shalom."

Many people claim to have heard the sound in meditation. I have been privileged to hear it on a number of occasions. It is absolutely amazing. It sounds like billions of voices chanting the "oon/uum/aum" sound, but not just chanting. It is as if the sound comes from every atom and even beyond the level of atoms, layer upon layer of sound arising from the very nature of everything in the universe, so that it has an amazing depth and resonance to it. It is impossible to describe, but after hearing it, I can see why it has been called the "Music of the Spheres." It is like the universe is continually singing itself into being.

Many of these mantras seem to be imitations of this Divine Sound, as if those who chanted them hoped to come into unity with that vibration. As you chant the mantra, and feel it vibrate in your whole body, you can also sometimes feel yourself resonating with the universe around you, especially if you "Practice the Presence" of God as you learned earlier, and chant the "Aum" at the same time, allowing the sound to penetrate everything around and in you.

However, it was not through repeating the mantra that I heard the sound. Rather, it was in the silence of the Prayer of Silence that I heard it. You may also hear the sound, as those things which keep you "out of tune" are cleansed from your life, and you begin to vibrate in unison with the energy of God.

In the book of Revelation in the Bible, there is an interesting passage which, for me, is related to more than just its metaphoric value. In Revelation 1:8 the *Christos* is quoted as saying, "I am the *Alpha* and the *Omega*, the beginning and the ending . . . which is, and which was, and which is to come, the Almighty." Two verses later, John says that, when he received his vision, he "was in the Spirit on the Lord's day." In other words, he was in a meditative trance when he saw the vision. We do not know the meditation practices he used, but the "*Alpha* and *Omega*" reference is very suggestive, especially considering all of the sharing of traditions and spiritual truths which took place in the Middle East at the time.

Of course, *Alpha* and *Omega* are the first and last letters of the Greek alphabet, so metaphorically they mean, "I am the beginning and the end," or "I am the Source of All and the goal of All."

But these words also suggest the "OM" or, in the form usually described in ancient texts, the "AUM." When you put the "A" of *Alpha* and the "OM" of *Omega* together, you end up with a mantra which starts with A and moves on to OM, sliding from A to OM, or AUM, just like the ancient texts describe. Did John meditate with the OM in order to enter into the state which gave rise to his visions?

It would seem that the Sound of the Silence may actually be "A-U-M."

It is interesting that when chanting "Shalom" – "SHAL-OM" -- the Hebrew word for peace and God's community, one is sounding out the same resonance as in "A-OM." The Arabic "Salaam," the greeting which means "Peace," has a similar effect. "Amen" also carries this sound.

The ancient writers claim that this is the sound of the universe and, in chanting it, the meditator is entering into the chorus which the universe makes. It is thus seen as the "seed" mantra from which all other mantras are built. One begins to wonder if, in the early Christian oral tradition which is lost, this was a key component in their meditative chants, especially when we have mantras like Abwoon, Amen, *Alpha* and *Omega*, and Shalom passed down to us.

Another interesting mantra from Tibetan Buddhism has uncanny similarities with some of Yeshua's teachings. The most important mantra of Tibetan Buddhism is "Om Mane Padme Hum" (pronounced "OM-Maa-Nay-Ped-May-Huum"). You can see the universal Om which introduces it. The Hum ending it is a resonant conclusion which again reverberates in the higher chakras when you chant it. But the "Mane Padme" is the interesting part in relation to Yeshua's teaching.

Yeshua speaks of the Kingdom of Heaven being like a jewel or pearl of great price for which we have to search. The Tibetan chant, "Mane Padme Hum" means that "the Jewel is in the Lotus." The "lotus of a thousand petals" is a symbol of the divine self, the Atman, which is similar to the *Christos*, the Divine Spirit, the Buddha Nature of which we have spoken before. The mantra says, in effect, that to find the jewel of great price, we need to look in the lotus which is the Atman/Spirit aspect of ourselves. That is where the Kingdom of Heaven really is. And the OM which is at the beginning of the mantra, is the sound of the Atman/Spirit continually singing itself into manifestation.

It seems that, in the mystical traditions of a number of religions, people have discovered essentially the same thing. When you begin to examine their discoveries about the Spirit, you realize they have perceived the same Divine Essence within everyone, whether they call it the Christ Nature or the Buddha Nature or the Atman. Differences of doctrine begin to fade away and unity, peace, compassion and love become much more important.

***

The Importance of the Meaning of the mantra

Of course, differences of doctrine and belief very quickly enter into all religions, and Christianity is no exception. The early history of the church is a history of conflicts over what was truth, and the arguments over truth ended up in the formulation of various competing doctrines which divided people and split empires. In the process, many mantras arose which reflect specific doctrinal positions.

Two popular, early mantras are still used widely today but, to me at least, suggest division and separation rather than unity. You need to be aware of what you meditate on, since the repetition of that which is negative can have profound consequences. We often use mantras in life without thinking about them, but now is the time to start examining the ones you use.

The two Christian mantras I find to be negative are, "Maranatha" and the Jesus Prayer, "Lord Jesus Christ, have mercy on me, a sinner."

In Aramaic, "Maranatha" means "Come Lord." It is the mantra which Fr. John Main and The World Community for Christian Meditation use centrally in their practice. This may seem like a good prayer on which to meditate, but you will be aware by now that I emphasize that God is always present with us. The purpose of entering the Silence is to become aware of the Divine Presence by removing those things which block it. What is wrong with "Maranatha" then, you may ask?

A mantra like "Maranatha," "Come Lord," repeated over and over, em-phasizes separation from God, not God's Presence. Whenever we enter the Silence, we ask for God's guidance, and we know God is always with us. But to continually say, "Come Lord," is like saying, "You are absent, Lord. I am ready for you to come, so please come now." If you continue to repeat it, you seem to be saying, "Why aren't you coming? I keep calling and you don't come." For this reason I find I cannot say that mantra because it denies the Presence I know is always with me.

I would suggest another mantra to put in place of that one. The mantra was taught to me in my inner learning and is, "I am in You: You are in Me." In this mantra, the meaning is all important. The "I" and the "Me" and the "You" are all interchangeable as God and us. God is saying to us, "I am in You: You are in Me." Then we are saying to God, "I am in You: You are in Me." This mantra reinforces the sense of union rather than the sense of sepa-ration, and practicing it while sensing God within us, and us within God, can be very powerful.

The Jesus Prayer arose within the same negative tradition of early Chris-tianity which produced "Maranatha." The Jesus Prayer, "Lord Jesus Christ, have mercy on me, a sinner," constantly emphasizes our limitations, our sinfulness and our separation from God, rather than the fact that God loves us and actively waits for us.

Of course, at some point we do have to realize our lives have been going in the wrong direction, repent and decide to turn our lives around and seek God's guidance, as in the story Yeshua told of the repentant Publican (Luke 18:10-14) which is the source of this prayer. We may even have to do this many times in our lives.

However, we do not have to continue reinforcing, many times a day, the idea that we are terribly sinful creatures. The Publican in Yeshua' story prays, "God be merciful on me a sinner," but then Yeshua says also, "this man went down to his house justified." He does not have to continue repenting over and over, every day, for the same errors. At some point, we have to accept God's forgiveness and move on to greater spiritual growth, without carrying a burden of guilt with us all the time.

Some people think that we have to keep asking for forgiveness for what they call, "Original Sin," which was inherited from Adam and Eve and is always with us. However, in Yeshua's teachings, and at the time he lived, there was nothing like the doctrine of Original Sin -- that was a much later development. Sins were errors of action, judgement or thought and, as in the story of Jonah and Nineveh, once they repented, people were forgiven. They did not have to carry the sins of the past, as was dictated in the later doctrine of Original Sin.

Every person is responsible for their own decisions and behaviour and, in the Silence with God, we can express our repentance, accept God's forgiveness and cleansing and move on to greater service, free of the weight of guilt.

Nor do we have to plead with God or with Yeshua to have mercy on us. God is always merciful. Like the father in the story of the Prodigal Son, God welcomes us back when we decide to come home (Luke 15:11-32). To continue asking for mercy is to deny that God hears the first time, and that God is always merciful.

Again, an alternate mantra, based on the Prodigal Son story, "God loves me: I am home," has a more powerful transformative effect than "have mercy on me, a sinner," which constantly reinforces our limits and denies God's continued love of us.

With any of these mantras, like "God loves me: I am home" or "I am in You. You are in Me," visualize the first half of the mantra moving from the base of the spine to the top of the head, and the second half from the head to the base of the spine. If you use "OM," repeat the OM going up and another OM going down, so you are surrounded by that one sound. That way you are surrounded by the mantra.

If you are deciding on a mantra, make sure you examine its implications carefully, because in repeating it hundreds, even thousands of times, you are reinforcing its message within your whole being and any negative implications will be magnified many times.

In modern writing on meditation, mantras are often called "affirmations," after the extensive work of Louise Hay on the subject. She and others have discovered in a very practical way that the words we repeat are the ones which affect us most. If we use negative words, we reinforce negative perceptions of ourselves and others. If we repeat positive, affirmative words, on the other hand, we learn to see the world and ourselves from a positive perspective.

We often say things like, "I am such a clutz," "I always make mistakes," "I hate those people," "I'm no good at anything," "I wish I hadn't been born." Louise Hay found that these negative phrases, used over and over, can have such negative effects that they can actually cause illness. She also found that just changing the negative phrases to positive "affirmations" about ourselves, can change our lives drastically, and can even lead to physical healing. This makes sense in terms of what we have discovered in the Prayer of Silence, because what we think is what we become. Affirmations can change our lives in profound ways.

Mantras, then, serve several purposes. The sound can be soothing, it can help us become aware of different centres in our bodies and activate them or can even connect us to the creative mystery of the universe. The mantra can also have profound meaning for us since it can carry us deep into the mystery of life and it can make positive change in our view of ourselves and others.

Experiments with school children have shown that, if they are told they are intelligent, they perform much better than if they are told they are stupid. Even water tastes differently if you put a jug on a paper with "Love" printed on it and another on a piece of paper with "Hate" printed on it. People have reported that the Hate-water even had a burning sensation in their mouths. Dr. Masaru Emoto has photographs in his books of water crystals which have been exposed to different words. They are a graphic illustration of the powerful effect of words on us and our environment, especially if repeated over and over, as mantras are.

One of the basic mantra in the Bible is that "God so loved the world" (John 3:16). With that as a base, all the other things fall into place. If what we repeat to ourselves denies the love of God, then we need to give that up, and seek God's interpretation of life, not the interpretation of various doctrines or arguments which make it obvious that those who formulated them did not believe in God's unconditional love.

***

Concentration

One other thing that mantras can do for us is to help us learn concentration. This is an aspect of mantras which is often spoken of in instructions for meditation. It is asserted that by spending hours concentrating on a mantra, always bringing our attention back to "just the mantra" or "just the breath," we develop discipline.

However, just sitting and chanting a mantra or concentrating on the breath can be very difficult, and many people give up meditation because it seems "boring and senseless" to them. And as I have said above, it also has the effect of keeping the focus on the speech centres of the brain, instead of allowing other aspects of awareness to develop.

That is why I have been taught a different approach to meditation, one which is designed to produce a progressive growth of awareness, self-knowledge and compassion. As you can see from what you have already accomplished, this is a more active approach to discovering the meaning of what is within and around you. You have learned concentration in the exercises in this book, but at the same time you have learned self-awareness.

The theory behind the Prayer of Silence is that it is better to develop concentration and awareness at the same time, with exercises which enrich all aspects of your life. Mantras may be able to deepen your concentration, and you may be able to enter into a variety of trance states as you become more proficient. But mantras should not be made into the centre of your practice.

I would suggest you continue to Practice the Presence of God around and in you, continue to resolve any difficulties which present themselves, and experiment with some of the simple mantras suggested here, if you want to see where they take you. Enter the Silence as usual, ask for guidance and then chant the mantra, surrounding your body with its energy.

Chapter Fourteen

Dealing with Dry Periods and "Dark Nights of the Soul"

Every once in a while I get phone calls saying, "Bruce. I seem to have gotten to a place where nothing is happening. I meditate and there isn't anything going on. What do I do?"

Most meditative traditions speak of "dry periods," when you sit in the Silence and nothing happens. These dry periods come occasionally on the spiritual path, sometimes even escalating into a variety of "Dark nights of the soul," as St. John of the Cross called them. There are different kinds of dry periods, which I will describe below, along with the reasons for them and things you can do to deal with them so that they do not prevent you from progressing further.

Since I cannot answer everyone's questions in person, this chapter is designed to address most of the problems you may run into.

***

Stagnation due to narrow concentration

People, who merely concentrate on a mantra or on the breathing or some other single point, often find that they get just so far on their path and then nothing seems to be happening for them. This occurs, not just with mantras, but also when you use only one method of growth while in the Silence. If you only concentrate on past lives, for instance, or psychic development or resolving emotional trauma, you will come up against a wall which blocks your progress. It is necessary to develop a well rounded and practical sense of how you are a reflection of the Divine in the world.

Some of Yeshua's followers obviously ran into this problem, because he advises, "Not every one who says to Me, Lord, Lord, shall enter into the kingdom of Heaven; but he who does the will of My Father in Heaven" (Mat. 7:21). All the repetitions of mantras or prayers or meditative techniques, repeating,

"Lord, Lord," over and over again, will not be sufficient to make you aware of God's Presence with you.

This phenomenon of dryness because of a narrow focus happens in all meditative traditions. The Tibetan Buddhists tell a story of one of their saints who spent twelve years meditating in a cave, trying to find enlightenment. Finally, he left in despair because his isolated meditations did not get him anywhere. He went into the market in the nearby town. There, he saw a dog which had been injured. He stooped down to help the dog and, in this act of compassion, finally found the illumination he was looking for.

In the same way, some people concentrate only on healing their physical ills. They will get to the point where, either all their ills are healed or, more likely, they will have some that cannot be healed for some reason and they will become discouraged. They have been spending all their time obsessed with health and sickness. This will soon lead to a dry period, because there is so much more in us that needs to be developed.

Also, if you only concentrate on beliefs or ideas or on relaxation or any of the other isolated aspects of the self, you will get to the point where you cannot go any farther with your practice. Only part of your being is involved in each of these things.

In order to overcome this kind of dry period, it is necessary to take a wider view of yourself. You are not just your body or your health. Nor are you just ideas. We started with the body in this book because that is the most obvious thing for most of us and because it is a way of finding a focus from which we can move to other areas. But we need to move beyond the body as well.

If you enter a dry period in your meditation because of a limited focus, try moving your awareness to another area of your total self. On the principle we have talked about before, that "you can always get anywhere else from here," any area you have made the centre of your meditation can lead to another area.

Perhaps the most important area to develop in attaining "perfection," is your relationship with other people. You need to examine your relationships with your family first, since that will teach you most about the roots of your personal relations, and then your friends, associates and even your enemies. You need to examine your memories and feelings as they relate to others, and then try to resolve any blockages you find there. This will quickly take you out of a dry period and start up your inner growth again.

We are not expected to withdraw from the world in order to attain our goal. It is precisely by being in the world that we find what we have attracted to ourselves by our beliefs and attitudes, and it is through examining our relationships that we begin to grow by understanding why all these people have been attracted to us.

If your dry period, caused by a narrow focus, persists, you may find that it is necessary to become involved in some form of service to others. This will help you to grow tremendously. Try volunteering some of your time to help others. In helping someone else, you will be extending yourself in very important ways, learning more about how you can relate to the world around you and, in the process, learning much more about yourself. In giving to others, you give even more to yourself, and you thus open the doors to greater inner growth.

***

Spiritual experience and dryness

Ironically, profound spiritual experience often leads to periods of dryness, when the effect of the experience "wears off" and we have to enter the "ordinary" world again. This has been the experience of many people, especially those who have Near Death Experiences or profound, life changing experiences of the Divine. Some people even go into severe depression after such an event.

As a result of your continued, regular meditation, or sometimes during times of crisis, you will have what have been called "Peak Experiences." You may have had these kinds of experiences already, since studies show that about 50% of people do have what they would call a "direct experience of the Divine." These are gifts to us to help us through to another stage of development.

We really can have a perception of the Divine when we strip away the things which block this perception, as we have been doing in the Prayer of Silence. Sometimes crisis situations provide this stripping away for us, but we can learn through regular meditation to enter more fully and regularly into these spiritual experiences.

But the crisis vision or the profound meditative experience, although giving us impetus for a while, does fade, partly because the blockages of our perception re-establish themselves.

I know a woman who had a profound Near Death Experience following a serious accident. She literally felt "held in the arms of God" and all her pain was taken away. It gave her inspiration for a while, but, as with many people, it took a long time to integrate the experience into her life. She often felt discouraged, because the experience gave her such a profound vision of what life could be, and then she was plunged back into all the usual troubles of life. After the NDE she became quite psychic and found she could do healing. She was able to move beyond the dry period in her development only when she started using those gifts to help others. This is often the case. You must put into practice what you have learned in these Peak Experiences.

Many people even become afraid of meeting God again. They are afraid of repeating the spiritual experience, ironically because they had such a wonderful sense of God's love and light and acceptance. There are a number of possible reasons for this.

The first is that, once they return to normal life, they begin to wonder if the experience was real. They actually begin to doubt their sanity. They begin to accept the world's definition of spiritual experience as illusion. So they are afraid to enter again into something which causes such conflict between the way most of their associates perceive the world, and the new way which is suggested by their spiritual experience.

Another reason people turn in anger against the memory of the spiritual experience is that they hoped the experience would absolve them of the responsibility to change their lives. They wanted God to do the work for them, and find instead that they still have to return to face the difficulties in spite of the experience.

That is a misunderstanding of the purpose of these experiences. They tell us that God loves us and that God is present with us. With that encouragement, we now have to start working to change our lives to get rid of other errors.

If you use some of the exercises in this book which are designed to correct errors, and take responsibility for your growth, your dry period will come to an end because you will see how you actually can take responsibility for your own spiritual growth, and that is very liberating. It opens up many possibilities to you.

And sometimes the difficulty we have with spiritual experience is just the contrast between the beauty of the spiritual experience and the ugliness and pain of the world to which we return. I know that was my experience.

As I have told you before, during a profound Near Death Experience as a young man, I was given the choice whether to come back to the body or not. I chose to return. It was my decision and I made it knowing full well that my body was very badly smashed up and required many months and years to recover. In spite of all that, after I returned to life, I often longed for the beauty of the NDE as an escape from the suffering I was going through. At times of great pain during my recovery, I regretted the decision I had made, and wished to return to the Light. I know firsthand the feelings which arise when we return to the body and its difficulties.

I did not realize that the suffering was part of the learning. I had to learn how to find my way to the enduring joy of the spiritual state, in spite of the suffering. The frequent dry periods in my own practice have been caused by that desire to escape the present. But we can never escape ourselves. We always have to live with who we are.

My learning has found its way into this book. I learned the hard way that what I needed to do was to concentrate in my meditation on the present, not try to escape the present. I had to get to know it, understand where I was "right now." I had to know my body, emotions, ideas, attitudes, relationships and actions NOW. And I had to do what I had contracted to do during that discussion on "the other side" – to teach the Prayer of Silence and write *The Thomas Book*. Only when I had written the books was I able to move on from that level to the next.

Many people think, "If only I could have an experience of God, then everything would be fine!" But they do not realize that the experience in itself is not sufficient for us. God does not suddenly change us with the experience, although the experience does open doors to other possibilities, doors which we can never shut.

I have found it necessary, not just to have spiritual experiences (however lovely they may be), but to work with the experiences in meditation – contemplate on them, read about others who have had similar experiences, open myself to other action of the Spirit, re-enter the memory of the experience in meditation and find out what it means in more depth.

If we have an experience of the Divine and then just leave it, it gradually becomes just a memory and fades into the past. Then the sense of nostalgia, even a very sad or despairing nostalgia, develops. In order to overcome the danger of turning the spiritual experience into mere nostalgia, it is necessary to re-enter the experience in the Silence and to learn as much as possible from it.

But how do you do this re-activation of the Vision? A method which draws on what you have already learned would be most helpful and that is what I suggest below.

***

Meditation Exercise: Re-entering spiritual experiences

Enter the Silence in the usual way. Then ask God to teach you why you experienced the Vision. Describe to God what you feel you experienced and how you feel about it – that is, bring your awareness up to date by recounting the whole thing to God.

This request for help and description of your understanding of the vision are important, because most spiritual experiences are given as a step along the spiritual path, and by entering into an exploration of the Vision, you are giving permission for God or your Guide to explain the lessons involved in the experience.

After this preparation, relax further, concentrate on the breathing and become aware of yourself as the Watcher, observing the breath. Once you have a sense that you have entered into the Watcher state of consciousness, re-enter the spiritual experience as you remember it. Visualize it as clearly as you can. Put yourself back into the place and time of the spiritual experience. Become aware again of what the Vision was, the feelings you had, who else was involved in the vision. Turn the vision from a past memory into a present experience.

Allow the Vision to speak to you again, but this time, once the Vision is in focus in the Silence, ask God or your Spiritual Guide to help you understand what you need to learn from the Vision. Be open to what arises. It may take several sessions in the Silence to understand what was involved in the Vision. In fact, there are usually many levels of meaning in spiritual experiences, so you will have to come back to this exercise from time to time to uncover the lessons which are there for you.

You will also find that the Vision is not just for your enjoyment. Explore what action or change needs to come about in your attitude to life, in your relationships, in your job. Does the Vision say anything about the direction you are taking in your life? Explore all of these things, because spiritual experiences are there to guide you to another level of growth if you will listen.

It is important to put into practice what the Vision suggests. This might involve studying, working with people, writing a journal in which you keep track of insights, writing a book, sharing the experience with others or even changing the whole direction of your life. Once you have re-activated the intent of the Vision and have started some action appropriate to what you discover, you will have brought yourself out of the dry period into a new process of growth.

***

The plateau effect

Another reason for dry periods is that, as we grow spiritually, we leave behind a lot of ego things (including beliefs) that made sense of our life in the past but which no longer speak to us. We have been letting go of our old personality and its errors bit by bit, but we haven't yet built up enough of a sense of the new dimension to know how it might give order and direction in our lives.

A story will put this in starker relief.

Imagine someone named Jim, who is in prison for murder. He decides to change, enters the Silence, and asks for God's help in turning his life around. In the process of time, Jim gradually eliminates the extreme anger and hatred which caused him to commit the murder in the first place.

The side effect of this change will be that he begins to lose friends, people who had been like him, filled with hatred and a desire for revenge. The change will be very difficult, because Jim cannot get away from the other prisoners, and a sense of violence and opposition constantly fills the air.

For a while, Jim will have no idea where the change in his personality is taking him. His former associates will ridicule him as a Holy Joe and may even abuse him physically to try to get him to return to their way of life. He will likely suffer intensely, not only from the outside, from the actions of the other prisoners, but also because his growing sense of compassion will cause him to feel guilt and remorse for what he has done in his life. He will also wonder why he decided on this spiritual path and will be sorely tempted to go back to his old, familiar ways.

But he will find that turning back is now impossible. He cannot get rid of the insights he has gained and he does not really want to stop his growth. He knows he has to go forward, however difficult it might be, even though at this time he does not know where he is going. He must ask for strength, realizing that there are many things he has to learn about his old life. Perhaps he will even have to find a way to atone for the pain he has caused all those other people who he has hurt.

This is what I call the "plateau period," the stage between the decay of the old ego and the coming into focus of the new Ego. And it may last for a short or long time depending on how much has to be done to resolve the errors of the past and to build up a new life free from the hatreds, fears and violence of the past.

Interestingly, this is a good account of what St. John of the Cross calls the Dark Night of the Senses. St. John discovered that on the spiritual path, we get to the point in our spiritual growth where the things of the senses, things which delighted us at one time, no longer interest us. We feel the sense of emptiness, but have not yet moved to the level where we can see clearly what the next phase of the spiritual life will involve.

To continue to grow, we must continue to enter the Silence on a regular basis and ask constantly for strength and guidance. We must let go of the errors which held us in the prison of the senses in the past, and gradually establish a relationship with the "God within" to discover the love and peace which can transform our life.

It is very important at this stage to try to do something about any hurt we have caused. This may involve contacting anyone we have injured or, if they are no longer around, we should look for a situation where we may be of benefit to others in similar circumstances. We must "reap what we sow," and if we sowed violence we must do something to heal violence if we are to be healed ourselves. This will seem like a dry period but is actually a time when the new person is in the process of forming.

This will take time, and Jim will have to persevere in his efforts. But gradually he will change, and in changing he will attract different people to him, likely other inmates who need help in their lives. Gradually, day by day, he will begin to develop a new personality, a new reason for being. He will have changed from a murderer filled with hatred to a compassionate man who can help others who are seeking meaning in their lives. Gradually, the new meaning in his life will emerge.

This is the actual process through which many former inmates, who have become prison, drug and prostitution councillors, have gone: they can help others because they have gone through the same difficulties themselves. They are what are called "Wounded Healers." Only those who have suffered the wounds of the inner being, and have found their way to healing, know how to guide others over the same path. This is why I am able to teach you about healing – because I have myself gone through a complex process of healing. Without that, all of my words would be merely theory.

***

Periods of transition

In a sense, Jim's story is an allegory of all of our lives. We are all prisoners to our old self and, as the old ego is left behind, for a while there will be little sense of what the new person will become. There are many transitional dry period.

In all of these dry periods, it is essential that we continue our practice of entering the Silence regularly, even when at times it seems that what we are doing is futile. Over many years of experiencing these alternating periods of growth and the plateaus in between, I have found that what is actually happening is that the process of meditation, prayer, reading, thinking and working with others is turning us into new people. It is deepening our ability to feel compassion, to perceive what is happening in and around us. We are gradually developing inner strength and the Spiritual Will through devotion and perseverance.

There can be many of these periods of growth. On the spiritual path, we tend to oscillate between periods of tremendous discovery and then periods when the death of the old way of perceiving makes life seem dry or even chaotic. Again, St. John of the Cross identified three of these Dark Nights, as he calls them: The Dark Night of the Senses, The Dark Night of the Soul and The Dark Night of the Spirit.

We have already seen that the Dark Night of the Senses is that period when sensual pleasures, ego pleasures, no longer attract us, and we are in the stage of transferring our loyalty from the senses of the body to the perceptions of the soul -- the religious feelings involved in theological ideas, music, devotion, art, beauty, service to others or literature.

The Dark Night of the Soul goes one step further. Those religious and artistic feelings which were central to your "religious" life lose their attraction. You do not respond to the sacred music or the chanting or the devotional practice anymore. Perhaps psychic things no longer interest you, if that was part of your religious development. You may have been devoting time to service to others, but you finally feel burned out and wonder what to do next.

If you have gotten that far, it means that you are ready to take the next great leap forward, but it looks like a leap into emptiness. That is because you are finally leaving behind even the religious feelings which gave you meaning in the past. Religion or art gave meaning, but they no longer offer any sense of meaning. If you do not know or believe there is anywhere to go from there, it is a difficult time indeed, because you think that you have reached the end of where there is meaning in life.

Now the universe seems to be meaningless or even hostile. You may even decide to become an atheist because, if religion is associated with God, and religion no longer seems to have any meaning, atheism seems the next logical step.

Finding your way out of the Dark Night of the Soul is very difficult, usually because you do not think there is anywhere else to go. You have not come to the conclusion that there is no God without a lot of inner searching and hard, often painful work. You consequently have a lot of attachment to that conclusion. It may not even seem necessary to move beyond the atheism or the anti-religious, anti-spiritual conclusions to which you have come. The only thing which seems to be left is materialism.

If you are willing to look at an alternative at that point – and I recognize that is not necessarily possible – then the Prayer of Silence is a way of getting through to another level of meaning. The Prayer of Silence offers the path of experience. It is the same path which materialism offers, except it offers exercises in which you can use your own consciousness to explore what is within you. It does not say to believe there is something there. Rather, it says to sit in silence and experience what happens to your consciousness as you become aware of your body or your emotions or other aspects of your inner nature.

The Prayer of Silence has some of the same difficulties with religion that the materialist has, in that it is not interested in doctrines and beliefs. In fact, it has arisen after both religion and materialism lost their meaning. It is the product of consciousness which has gone through the Dark Night of the Soul and has found something else. It wants evidence in the form of confirming experience. But instead of looking for confirmation in the outer world, it tests everything to see if it is actually reflected in the inner consciousness.

In many ways I went through the Dark Night of the Soul after the Near Death Experience. I was going to be a Christian minister, but that did not make sense any more. I attended church, but found it increasingly meaningless, until I got to the point just after writing *The Thomas Book*, where I no longer went to church. I knew there was some other meaning within me, but had not yet formulated what it was. In many respects, even with all my spiritual experience, I was a materialist. It was the Prayer of Silence which made it possible for me to move on to the next stage.

The witness of many people who have taken this path over the centuries is that, if you persist in your inner search, you will move beyond religious belief and doctrine to "spiritual" discoveries. You will enter into *Gnosis*.

The Dark Night of the Spirit is the hardest of all, but when you persevere, it leads to the most profound level of spiritual growth. To become "one with God," you must give up attachment to everything else, and that is very difficult to accomplish.

The Dark Night of the Spirit often involves the death of someone near to you or the loss of a job or the end of a relationship on which your world depended. Encephalitis was my Dark Night of the Spirit because it seemed to destroy all meaning. In it I lost everything – ego, job, position in society, memory, reputation. Fortunately, my wife and family stood by me as I worked through that tremendous loss, but mostly the struggle is internal in this phase of spiritual growth. I had to depend on what I had learned in my earlier spiritual practice. I had to put it all to use to find how it applied to healing this most drastic of losses. It involved faith in God, even when everything that had happened seemed to suggest that the universe was meaningless, or even actively vindictive.

However, out of the death of the old person, and out of all the suffering, a new person emerged. The Dark Night of the Spirit is told graphically in the Book of Job in the Bible, where Job loses everything, but refuses to "curse God and die."

The sense of the Divine Union which arose from my experience of the loss of everything, was worth it all, however. I describe that experience in the last chapter of this book.

It was worth it all. Yet at the time, all that held me on the path was faith, and the accounts of others that there was something on the other side of the

darkness, which is why I tell you about my experience, so that you can persevere as well, if you are going through suffering.

I read the Book of Job many times during the period of my illness. His
words were like a protest, the protest I also made:

> *For I know that my Redeemer lives,*
> *And He shall stand at last on the earth:*
> *And after my skin is destroyed, this I know,*
> *That in my flesh I shall see God.   (Job 19:25-26)*

I had practiced the Prayer of Silence for many years by the time I got the
encephalitis, I had written the gospel portion of *The Thomas Book* and had
spent many years talking with Yeshua in meditation, so I knew that there had
to be something to work toward, even if the darkness of that time seemed to
deny that there was any meaning.

It was important to me at that time to assert my belief in reincarnation,
if only for my own sanity, because our culture usually thinks of people with
disabilities as "damaged goods." And if you are an academic, whose life has
drawn its meaning from the brain and its knowledge, and your memory is
wiped out, it seems like there cannot possibly be any meaning left in life. But
having experienced past life recall, I knew this was not the only life I had. For
some reason, this part of this life led to a loss of memory, but I knew, deep
within, that not all of my being was negated just because one life seemed to
have come to a dead end. This life was only part of a larger spiritual whole, and
I had to find the reason why it had ended up as it did.

And I knew, because of this passage, that Job also believed in reincarnation, and that even if my body was destroyed before I found God in this
lifetime, even if my "skin is destroyed," still, "in my flesh I shall see God."
I will return, even if I die. That assertion of continuing life in other bodies,
in which I could search for God, was a great comfort when this body was so
badly damaged. And I finally knew that my goal was clear: "in my flesh I
shall see God."

It is very rare, St. John of the Cross says, for people to have the courage to
persevere through these Nights to the rewards beyond them, and I can see why.
But now that you know about them, if they do come your way, you can endure
them and move into the profound spiritual perception which is beyond.

It is important to keep going. This is where faith and trust come in. This is what Søren Kierkegaard spoke of in his book *Fear and Trembling.* Faith is being able to step into the darkness, knowing that solid ground will be there for our feet to stand on in spite of the fear and trembling we feel as we move through the difficult times in our lives. This is a matter of trust that the inner guidance, which has guided us this far, will be faithful in taking us forward to the next step in our growth. Patience and faith are the keys here.

This is also why I have led you gradually through the development of your inner awareness, so that you know from experience that, when difficulties arise, you can keep going and find meaning beyond the inner darkness. Bring everything into the Silence and it can be cured. You now have the meditation exercises which can address almost all issues in your life.

The story of the Hebrew slaves delivered from bondage in Egypt by Moses can be seen as an allegory of this process. We are all slaves in our old life, in "the flesh pots of Egypt." Deliverance is very seldom into a Promised Land. Rather, we have to wander in the wilderness for quite a while until the old generation (the old personality) has died off. Then we can enter the Promised Land as new people.

It is often only when we look back that we see what has been happening and that there has actually been direction in what seemed like aimless wandering. But it does take work and devotion to keep from falling back into the old way of seeing things, the old ego orientation which would like desperately to keep us from changing.

***

Darkness and the blockage of fear

I have found from working with others that what I call, "darkness and the blockage of fear," is a fairly common cause of dry periods. It is actually like a wall which seems to stop you in your tracks. It comes after you have progressed quite far on the spiritual path.

When this dry period comes, you will often sense, with an unconscious yet powerful fear, that something is about to emerge from your memories which you do not want to face. You do not know what you fear, but the fear is so powerful you do not want to go any further.

When these fear-based dry periods arise in your time in the Silence, it is very difficult to move forward. You may start making excuses to stay away from your regular meditation practice. You may even take on so many re-sponsibilities on the job or in the community that you have no time left for the Silence -- but this is just avoidance. Unfortunately, this is how many people come to the end of their meditation practice, because they do not deal with the unconscious fear.

To understand what is happening, it is important to be aware of something about the personality at this point. As we become more aware in meditation of who we really are – the Atman/Spirit which is expressed as the Watcher in our everyday life -- we gradually let go of our material egos and the things of the body and allow the truly eternal aspects of ourselves to form a spiritual Ego around the Watcher, the Atman/Spirit.

However, I have discovered through experience that a strange thing hap-pens in the more advanced levels of spiritual growth, and this strange thing is directly related to the contrast between the Ego and the ego.

If you have been following the exercises in this book, at the same time as you have been getting rid of negative aspects of the ego, you have also been building positive aspects of consciousness (love, compassion, joy, kindness, generosity, etc.) into a coherent spiritual Ego with which you relate to the world around you. This Ego arises from the divine centre of your being and has great strength because it is connected to the divine creative centre. In creat-ing this Ego, you are forming what is called "God-consciousness" or "Christ Consciousness."

When you encounter the remaining negative proto-personalities in medi-tation at this stage of spiritual development, the contrast between the positive Ego and the negative ego can make you feel you are confronting concentrated evil, *emerging from somewhere in yourself.* It can be very frightening to think that this is actually coming from you. You may even wonder if you are evil or are being influenced by evil, even though it is merely the remnants of your old ego. You may sense darkness or intense anger or hatred or violence in some area of your body or emotional/intellectual field. You will also sense that this dark area resists the movement of the Watcher through it. This darkness, stored in the *theta* frequencies of the brain, even takes on symbolic character-istics, so that it becomes whatever you think of as evil – Satan, devils, aliens or some other evil creature. It seems to be something which is actively opposed to the Divine awareness which is developing in you.

Something else may happen at this advanced stage as well and, although you will likely not run into this experience, it is good to be prepared by being aware that it is a possibility. Most spiritual traditions are aware of what they call discarnate negative "spirits," the ghostly remains of people who have died in violent ways – gang wars, murders, executions or other deaths which free the negative emotions from the body, but which are no longer attached to the soul which has gone into the higher spiritual realms or has been reincarnated. Just like the proto-personalities, which are the fragments of our disintegrated ego, these "bhutes" as they are called in India, are not complete people, but they are capable of expressing themselves through the lower emotions, especially if a living person gives them a "home." These "spirits" often seek embodiment in living people who have attracted them through their own intensely negative thoughts. In this way violent people find their own violent tendencies augmented by these "psychic remains."

However, not only negative people experience these things. All advanced spiritual beings, like Yeshua or Buddha, must go through the process of facing these tempters. Yeshua met his temptations in the wilderness. Buddha faced his temptations under the Bo tree. Martin Luther wrote of his experience of throwing an ink pot at the Devil and, as we have already noted, Jung found that we all have to face our personal devils at some point if we are to be whole.

The fear which arises from these negative sources, whether in the self or in other beings, can be so great -- if you are ignorant of its source -- that you may enter into a dry period or even stop your growth entirely because you do not want to face them. What do you do to get rid of this fear?

***

Meditation Exercise: Getting rid of the darkness

Enter the Silence as usual. Ask God to help you realize who you really are and to help you overcome the errors which prevent you from being whole.

Once you have relaxed the body and are concentrating on the breathing, imagine yourself, as the Watcher, moving away from the body and looking back at the body. This may take some practice but, if you have been doing the exercises in this book, you will likely be able to do it fairly easily by now. Sense in this process that, although the body is important, you are actually independent of the body and the ego connected with the body. Keep doing this in your times in the Silence until you achieve a sense of separation of the Spiritual Self, the Watcher, from the body and ego.

Once you have been able to do this, move your awareness to the part of your body in which you sense the fear or anger or hatred or other negative feeling. It could be anywhere from your toe to your head, but is often in some part of your chest or abdomen because this is where the ego manifests many of the negative emotions on which is builds its world.

Do not feel fear. Recognize that you are not dealing with evil itself, but only with a manifestation of the negative which is left in your fragmented ego or the fragmented ego of someone else who seeks to intrude into your life.

If you withdraw your consciousness from the body to the Watcher, you will find something interesting happens to the ego and its manifestation in the body. The ego will actually seem to become independent of you, the Watcher, and the ego can even speak to you through the inner voice. Within its limits, it is a complete personality. Encourage it to talk. Let it speak its concerns, its fears, its angers or sense of being attacked or threatened.

Do not contradict it. In fact, it helps to agree with it in a sympathetic but detached way so that it does not feel threatened and it feels free to talk. It is a personality fragment but is as complete as some people, so it can talk quite coherently if you let it. Let it express all its concerns, but do not take those concerns onto yourself. It may become angry and even swear at you. Remember, it was part of your ego in the past and, in your earlier life, it likely had a prominent role to play in your relationships and in the world you built around you. Now you know you no longer want it to be part of you so, once it has said what it wants to, decide definitely that you want to let it go.

From the perspective of the Watcher, tell God you want to grow beyond the limited perspective of this personality fragment within you. Ask God to cleanse all the error of this ego fragment from you. Then breathe twelve times in your meditation, each time feeling the divine cleansing air coming in with the in breath and the negative blockage gradually leaving with the out breath.

If this fear or blockage has been with you for some time, you may find it exists in layers, so that you have to go through a series of meditations where you identify each related ego fragment in your body, allow it to speak in order to bring it into the open, and then ask God for cleansing. If a similar fragment, from deeper in your ego, emerges a month later or even years later, go through the same process. Gradually, you will be able to move beyond the dry period caused by this blockage and will then be able to continue with your growth.

There is reason to believe that many cases of Multiple Personality Syndrome are caused by these ego fragments which have been suppressed for a long time and have taken on a life of their own. In a sense, we all have multiple personalities. Just think of how you can be an angry person at one time, a loving person at another and a fearful person at yet another. This is because you are still controlled by these ego personality fragments. As you cleanse them from you, gradually you will become more integrated and whole. Instead of being an ego, you will become an Ego, an expression of the unity which is God.

***

Keep going

Mark Twain said, "If you're going through Hell, keep going." Good advice. Do not stop in your own Hell but keep going till you get out of it.

When you come to a dry period in your practice, keep going with your regular meditation. The suggestions above may help you identify some of the causes of the blockage and they will give you a sense of how the personality functions during the process of spiritual growth. But sometimes you just need to allow time to heal and change you. So, keep going with your practice. Continue to enter the Silence, even if nothing seems to be happening. Relax, ask for God's guidance, withdraw to the Watcher and sense the breath flowing in and out of your body. Sense the Presence of God in and around you. Continue doing this even if "nothing seems to be happening." Something is happening deep within you, and as you continue with this, you will find that whatever is forming within you will gradually find expression in some area of your life.

You sometimes have to demonstrate that your devotion is not just all words and that you actually do want to change and become whole. Sometimes these dry periods are actually periods of testing to see if you have the strength and perseverance to go on to the next stage. You have to persevere, to learn patience and inner strength before you will be allowed to enter the next stage of the spiritual journey.

This is often a way to protect you as well. If you are not ready or have not developed the required abilities, you would be hurt very badly if you were allowed to proceed farther along the path of spiritual development. Some things can only be healed when you have developed the required inner perception, wisdom and strength. Have patience. The Inner Divine Guide knows what you need.

One quotation which I have found very helpful in getting through many difficulties, including dry periods, is

> In all your ways acknowledge Him,
> And He shall direct your paths. (Prov. 3:5-6).

I have a little plaque with that quotation, sitting on my dresser. It was a gift to me after my fall down the shaft in 1966. Meditating on that mantra during times of tremendous pain and disorientation has been very helpful, because it has kept me centred and has given me direction.

Chapter Fifteen

"*I am in You. You are in Me.*" -- *The Gift of Divine Union*

"I and My Father are One." (John 10:30)

This final chapter is about the aims of the Prayer of Silence, the goal toward which we strive. The Prayer of Silence is different from most meditation systems, as you have likely already discovered. Most systems of meditation teach that we must transcend our humanity and become pure spirit. The Prayer of Silence teaches that we become spiritual as soon as we become "fully human."

As you are aware, we do not aim to destroy ego. In fact, we have attempted to transform ego from its selfish orientation to one which is united with all people and with the universe and God. The ego gradually becomes Ego as it changes its focus.

The Prayer of Silence also avoids suppressing any fears or hatreds or other negative feelings or attitudes or ideas. Instead, it brings these things actively to the surface of consciousness in order to transform them. We do not avoid the darkness within us, through the use of mantras, drumming, chanting or other devices designed to suppress the contents of the mind. Rather, we actively enter into the inner darkness, understand it and correct the errors we find there. Again, the aim is not to escape from "the things of the world" into a state of bliss, but rather to allow our inner problems to be transformed, so that hatred becomes love, fear becomes faith, anger becomes harmony. The final result is that we do not escape into bliss: Bliss becomes us.

Perhaps that is the key to what the Prayer of Silence is. Most spiritual philosophies are dualistic, in that they think there is a battle between the good and the evil, reality and illusion, Heaven and Hell, light and darkness or some other duality. "Evil" is usually identified in these philosophies with the body or the physical world or our desires and passions. Because money, sex and other desires are identified with both the body and the passions, they are especially condemned by most spiritual traditions.

This is where the Prayer of Silence is radically different. "Radical" means "from the roots." The very root of the ideas in the Prayer of Silence is different from most spiritual teachings. The Prayer of Silence sees the world as completely real and completely good. And in the Prayer of Silence there is no division between the world and God. In fact, it teaches that the world is a manifestation of God. Right down to the atoms and sub-atomic particles, the world arises from God. How can atoms, and things made of atoms, be evil?

And this goodness extends to all we are. The body is good. The desires are good. The ego is good. It is as the book of Genesis in the Bible says, "Then God saw everything that He had made, and indeed it was very good" (Gen. 1:31).

Then where does what appears evil come from? Haven't we been learning to be Dwellers in Two Worlds? Is not one of them good and the other evil?

In the Prayer of Silence, there are two worlds only because our minds, looking on the one world which has arisen from God, can see two worlds. Our minds create the division between truth and error. In the Prayer of Silence, evil is actually only ignorance and error. When we understand, when we achieve *Gnosis*, when we correct the error, then what appeared to be "evil," disappears. It arose in the mind and, when the mind changes, it is no more. Because of this, the only thing that needs to be changed is our mind, our way of seeing the world. Once we transform that, as we have been doing in all the exercises in this book, then we are able to realize the unity between us and the world and God.

That is why forgiveness is so important. We say for convenience that God forgives us our sins, but actually God never condemned us. God is like the father in the story of the Prodigal Son. God waits on the road for us to return. God does not require that we be punished or that someone else be punished in our stead. God merely waits for the Son to change his mind and return home where he is welcomed into the family which was always waiting for him to return. Nor were there ever any "sins." Sin is only the result of ignorance. Once we know what is in harmony with God and choose that way, then what was sin disappears. Neither the body nor the world was the cause of "sin." Only ignorance kept us from being aware of the Presence of God, which has always been around us and within us. The Kingdom of God is always within us. Once we know where to look, we can find it. The Prayer of Silence merely teaches us where to look.

You have learned to enter the Silence of God, to feel the Divine Presence around you, to see God in others and in the world. Even your ego, your sense of "I am," has changed. Instead of feeling identity with the body or possessions or social position, you have gradually begun to realize that your true identity lies in the "things of the Spirit," in love and joy and peace and generosity and compassion. Body and possessions and social position are not evil and you do not try to destroy them. All you do is discover where the true values lie. You change your priorities.

Some of you have even begun to get a sense of how God can be present in your own life and in your relationships. You may even be able to talk to God, as a person talks to his/her friend. You can see how God is in other people and that, as Yeshua said, "Inasmuch as you did it to one of the least of these My brethren, you did it to Me" (Matt. 25:40). This statement gives us a profound responsibility because it means that, whatever we do, we ultimately do to God.

Have we come to the end of what the Prayer of Silence offers, then? Is there anything else you can aim at besides continuing with your practice and gradually growing until you are conscious of your oneness with God? Actually, there is and there is not.

Whatever else we do is just adding onto what we have already discovered. We refine our practice, we resolve any other difficulties, we seek to integrate all aspects of our Self so that we function as a unity instead of as conflicting parts and we seek to develop more of the intimacy of our relationship with God so that, like Yeshua, we can know God as Abba.

However, we can take another of the sayings of Yeshua and work actively toward achieving what he achieved. We can seek the unity which Yeshua claimed to have found when he said, "I and My Father are one." Not only do we look for God in the world and in others, not only do we seek to serve others to help them in their lives, and not only do we seek to perfect our inner being to reflect what we know to be the nature of God in love, joy, peace and other positive values -- we also seek the experience of Oneness. This is what is called the Christ Consciousness, the realization in our own selves that we are one with "the God force" in the universe.

How do we do that?

We looked at the meaning of *Gnosis* earlier in this book. In some ways you have already developed your own *Gnosis*, your inner knowledge of God. But when Yeshua said, "I and My Father are one," (John. 10:30) he was indicating that there is something else we can try to achieve in our relationship with God. Later in John's Gospel, Yeshua is reported to have said further in his prayer to God before his death, "And the glory which You gave Me I have given them, that they may be one just as We are one. I in them, and You in Me, that they may be made perfect in one . . ." (John. 17:22-23). Yeshua obviously wanted his disciples to find the same union with God which he experienced, the same experience of "glory," of bliss which comes with Divine Union.

The next question, of course, is, "How do we develop an awareness of this Oneness?"

Perhaps it is not right to say that we can "develop" this added feature of our relationship with God. For most people who have experienced it, this next step was a gift from God, something which arose from their continued practice of all aspects of the transformation of the Self through the Prayer of Silence or another spiritual practice.

There is no guarantee that we will be given this gift of oneness, but as you continue with the exercises I have outlined in this book, you will gradually develop a greater sense of union with God, the world and those around you. You will find a deepening sense of the Presence of God within and around you as well, and that will itself bring a sense of union. You may already have experienced the profound Love and Joy which arise from deep within you, and are so wonderful they are almost painful -- when you can only say to God, "I love You," because nothing else seems appropriate. That will arise from the continued practice of the Prayer of Silence.

However, there are a couple of things which can help toward the sense of union with God. It requires first of all a transformation of your whole moral being so that the things you do and say and think move you toward complete harmony rather than disharmony. Remember, in as much as you do anything to others, you do it to God, because everything that is, is an expression of the Divine Nature. That will bring you to greater harmony.

***

Meditation Exercise: The perception of oneness

In most cases, when we meditate, we focus on "something," whether it is on our day, on relationships, on ideas or beliefs or fears, on the Presence of God with us, or some "thing" else. These are all meditations on "something" because we seek to develop spiritual focus and it is very difficult to meditate on nothing. It is even difficult to see how meditating on nothing could possibly help us. If we meditate on union with God, is not that something?

In fact, meditating on nothing is the hardest thing to do. There is a way to do it, however, and there is a reason for doing it as well. This also is part of the Prayer of Silence.

It has been said that God is not actually in the things around us, but in the spaces between all the things of our life. God is not actually in our beliefs or fears, in our relationships or possessions. God is not even in bodies and atoms and sub-atomic particles. These are all "things" which have arisen from God, as we have seen before. But, as the Jewish mystics say, God is really "Ain Soph," "No Thing." This next step involves focusing on No Thing.

As usual, in order to do this, you need to enter the Silence, relax, ask for God's guidance and Presence, move to the Watcher consciousness and become aware of the body and all its parts. Move your consciousness from one part to another. It is through the body, as usual, that we become aware of the aim of this meditation.

But just stop a minute, because I have to do something different here. I found it very difficult to describe what you should do in this exercise, so instead of the usual instructions, I decided to enter into the state of union myself, and from that state I typed into the computer what I saw and how I thought you could get there by following my words. Read over these instructions a number of times to become aware of what is there, and then you will be able to follow my words.

These words come to you from the Silence, beyond the world of things.

As I sit in meditation, trying to figure out how to describe this aspect of your spiritual path, I realize that what I am experiencing is beyond words, even beyond the parables which Yeshua used to point the way to the Kingdom of God. Somehow, this step does not even lend itself to expression with parables.

Some people say that Ain Soph is like the well from which the water of life flows, but then this makes of Ain Soph, a well, which is not No Thing. We can think of Ain Soph as Source, but even then we have the sense of a place from which all things flow.

Notice that here I am trying to describe the place or condition of Being from which "things" come. As I type, my awareness is in the state beyond things. I type these words from that experience, and try to give you an idea of where I am and how I got here.

Can we actually experience this Source? Actually, we can, but it requires that we enter into the experience, not into thoughts or ideas or even visualization, even though that has been valuable in our search, because all of these are "things."

It is time to enter into the Silence in your usual way. Relax, ask for God's guidance, focus on the breathing and then gradually withdraw to the Watcher. From the perspective of the Watcher, move your awareness over your whole body. Become aware of its totality by moving your attention over and through your whole body.

Once you have become aware of the whole body, move your awareness to the body as parts – legs, arms, hands. Then, move your awareness behind your head, so that you are aware of your head in front of you.

Once you have done that, move your awareness to the ears, eyes and mouth. Become aware of all these levels of division, from your whole body to your head to the parts of your head. Do not rush. You are becoming aware of "things" so that you will be able to move your awareness beyond the level of things.

From ears and eyes, move your awareness to perceive the cells which make up the ears and eyes. Focus on the eyes and the cells in the eyes. Be aware of each individual cell. Sense the cells and their interactions as they form and sustain the life in your body.

From there move your awareness to the molecules which make up the cells. Notice, we are moving to smaller and smaller parts of the body. Choose one cell and sense the movement of the molecules within that cell. It might help to check a reference work or the internet to see what cells and molecules look like, so that you can do this exercise more realistically.

After this, refine your view even further. Sense the atoms which make up the molecules. We are getting down to the smallest units of manifestation which make up what we think of as "the world." But there are still sub-atomic particles we can see within the atoms. Visualize those sub-atomic particles whirling in their orbits, as you move your awareness to smaller and smaller areas of awareness.

With the sub-atomic particles you perceive the smallest aspects of "things" that we know of. But we want to go even further than that. We want to move beyond "things" to another kind of awareness entirely.

At this stage, it is time to let go even of these smallest of "things" and to enter into the space between the smallest particles and energy clusters. Allow your awareness to enter into the spaces between atoms. This is where I am waiting for you to show you the way into this deep Silence.

You will find that this inner space is almost infinite. The atoms take up such a small amount of the space available that, when you perceive them accurately, it will seem as if the atoms are whirling around silently like stars in the night sky. And we are here, the Watcher, aware of the darkness of interatomic space, seemingly alone. Spend some time being aware of this space and the feelings you have here. This is not just "visualization." The Watcher can actually enter into this space and, when you do, the effects are profound indeed.

As I write these words on the keyboard, I am in this space with the atoms like stars. I am channelling the words out of this amazing infinite space between all the atoms.

As you concentrate on the space, you will actually begin to sense the Presence, the God Force, from which all the atoms arise, and from which all the "things" in your life arise. This is the space of the Zero Point Field we spoke of earlier, the place where there is nothing, yet the space which is full of intense activity.

This place is without "things" but it is full of consciousness. Here our consciousness is one with the Consciousness which unites and gives rise to all that is. You will begin to discover that you, the Watcher, are not one of the "things" in the universe. You have gone beyond things to something else – to pure awareness. You will also find that you are not separate from the Consciousness of the Universe, which actually is this space, but you are one with this infinite Consciousness. Space and Consciousness are one here.

If you stay here in meditation long enough, you will sense "absolute oneness" because your being and the Being of God are One. There is no separation here because you are no longer an object, a thing. You are now pure consciousness and you can be one with the Consciousness of God, beyond objects, beyond actions, beyond things. Those who have experienced this oneness refer to it as being like a drop in the ocean. There is no separation between the drop and the ocean.

Stay here for a time, feeling yourself within the Root from which All arises, but which is independent of all those things. Stay here in the Absolute Silence for a time each day, and you will enter into a Peace and Love and

Joy and Bliss which are always available, because they are the Source from which the universe arises. You share the same consciousness which is the Consciousness of God. This is Nirvana, because here all things and the desire for all things is "blown out."

I am writing these words while in this state of Oneness with God. It is hard to bring myself to type the words into the computer, but I can do that knowing that deep within me the Oneness with God is not disturbed. The words arise from the Silence only to guide you to follow them into this amazing Silence and Bliss.

When you are here, you do not want to leave, to go about the acts of the day, because they seem so trivial, so divorced from the ultimate reality which is here in the infinite Silence and darkness – a special kind of darkness which is even before light came into being.

I can hear the world around me, but here, at the Centre, is such peace that it is tempting to stay here, always. Why would one want to leave? Why would one want to seek embodiment? Why would one want to be incarnate when this Bliss is here, waiting within me? Then I know that it does not matter that I have a body. This Bliss is always here, within, just like the Kingdom of God is always within us and around us.

I now know that it is possible to stop the events of the day at any time, enter into the Silence and the awareness of the Watcher and then to withdraw, smaller and smaller, until I arrive at the awareness of Pure Consciousness beyond the manifest world.

Sit and experience it as long as you wish.

Here there is no time and no rush.

[After you have done this exercise a number of times, and have had some success in entering into the spaces between "things," you can move your awareness a step further. You can actually will yourself to move to the time before the universe of things came into being. The memory of that time is there within us all, and within the spaces of the Divine Silence, of a time when there were no things but only the movement of consciousness, because we are, indeed, one with God. You can will your Being into a time before time, when the Presence of God moved upon the waters of consciousness, moving in a circular motion, before there was any material substance to take form, moving in a Consciousness that would manifest eventually as the universe in its many levels of being. But this is an indication of what you can do sometime when you are ready. Do not rush this either.]

And when you are ready to return to ordinary consciousness, just wiggle your fingers and toes, become aware of the physical body, within which you manifest your infinite consciousness, and open your eyes to see the world of things in a new light. Know that within all those things you see around you, is this infinite Ain Soph, from which everything arises and to which everything returns. Know also that you do not have to wait until the end of time to return here, to the Divine Source, because you now know how to return to the Beginning any time you want. Here is to be found Infinite Peace.

As you practice this meditation, you will also become aware how your mind actually builds the world you experience. Edgar Cayce often said, "Mind is the builder."

As you change your mind and bring it into harmony with the Divine Mind, you will live more and more in a world of harmony because that is the world you will build.

***

I wrote the above while in that state of Bliss. It is impossible to describe, but perhaps reading that, and then practicing the exercise yourself, you will begin to discover the state of consciousness which is beyond our manifest identity, and beyond the things with which we surround ourselves. There you will find union with God.

***

Contemplation Exercise: The gift of Divine Union

There is another kind of union which we can experience, but this is a union which is more a gift than something we can develop or enter into through a particular meditation exercise.

Yeshua said, "I and My Father are one." This statement has been turned into doctrines by the churches, where they argue about how Jesus and God could be one. Was he of the same "substance" as the Father, or was he of a different "substance"? Was Jesus actually God, or was he an expression of God? How was he related to the Holy Spirit? And how was the Holy Spirit related to the Father? Are the Father, Son and Holy Spirit actually three equal aspects of the one God? Are they a Trinity? Or are these metaphors for how we can know God, where God is made known as a Father, as the Holy Wind, as the incarnate Son? Wars have been fought over these questions and countless people have been killed, tortured and burned at the stake because of their beliefs about these questions. They are by no means trivial.

But, interestingly, when you come back from the experience in the above exercise, of oneness with God, with Ain Soph, with the infinite Consciousness and Bliss which you find in the spaces between all the things of existence, you realize that Yeshua was speaking of an experience in which we can all participate. We, too, can be one with God.

In claiming that "I and My Father are one," Yeshua was drawing on an ancient tradition. From the very first, the biblical text asserts that human beings are in the image of God, are in some sense One with God (Gen 1:26) and therefore it is not blasphemy to seek to experience that Oneness. Yeshua went further by saying that this Oneness with God can be applied to other people. Yeshua taught that "the Kingdom of God is within you," in the same way that the Father was in him.

In case anyone had any doubts about whether Yeshua was including others in this Oneness, John's Gospel asserts that Yeshua said, after the resurrection, "I am not yet ascended to my Father: but go to my brethren and say to them, I ascend unto my Father and your Father, and to my God and your God" (John 20:17). This is not just Yeshua's Father or Yeshua's God. This is the God and Father of all people. Thus, John's message concludes where it began, where it said of Yeshua that "as many as received him he gave the power to become the Sons of God" (John 1:12). Yeshua said that everyone was able to become a "Son of God," one with God.

Sometimes the experience of oneness arises as a gift, not as the result of an exercise in meditation, although they both have their own validity. The experience of oneness in meditation can be repeated and we can return to it as often as we wish. The experience which is a gift has a different quality to it and must be accepted as a gift. It cannot be repeated unless it is given to us again.

A few years ago I had such a gift which speaks of the union between Atman/Spirit and God, between us and the Source of our being. I hope it will give you at least a small feeling of another place this Prayer of Silence can take you. I know that I am not the only one who has had this experience. It is a gift that many people have had and is a great blessing. But do not feel that unless you have this gift, you have come up short on the spiritual path.

Actually, all traditions warn against striving only for these experiences, what St. John of the Cross calls "spiritual gluttony," or the Eastern traditions call "Siddhis." To seek only an experience, however profound, is to lose sight of the ultimate instruction to "Seek first the Kingdom of God and His righteousness and all these things will be added to you" (Matt 6:33).

Sometimes these experiences are described as the aim of the spiritual life, but they are not. Our search does not end there, but continues as we draw closer to God and to our fellow human beings in our daily meditation and in our service to others. In a sense, "spiritual experiences" are a brief amplification of what we can find regularly in the Silence in our daily practise. You might want to ask God for this gift sometime, without being attached to it.

***

But let me tell you the story.

It was a lovely summer day, August 3rd, 1997. We were camping in a place called Kenosee, in south eastern Saskatchewan, Canada, about a two hours drive from where we live in Regina. It was a lovely, warm afternoon and we went down near the lake and sat on blankets spread on the grass under the pine trees. My wife was reading, my daughter was drawing and I was reading the works of an ancient Greek philosopher, Plotinus.

As I read Plotinus, I became aware of how complex his logic was, how sharp the intellectual distinctions were which he was making, how he was trying to define his subject with minute exactness. Then I became aware how my own intellectualism, in spite of many years of meditation and prayer and cleansing, was hard and sharp and often angry at times. I could almost feel the hardness and separation and sharpness of my own ideas as something tangible. So I put the book down and lay back on the blanket and entered the Silence to find out about this aspect of my mind and how it functioned and interpreted things. It is interesting that Plotinus had the Unitive Experience several times in his life and longed to have it again.

Once I had entered the Watcher consciousness, so that I could become aware of the patterns of my thinking, and could experience the nature of my thought more accurately, and once I had brought my ideas into focus as much as I could, I realized that I did not really want to think that way. It was an almost angry way of thinking and I sought something more gentle than I had been practicing. So I let go of all the separations and divisions and asked God to cleanse the error in my intellectual approach. Then I lay there with my eyes closed, letting the error go and feeling it wash from me with the breath.

When I opened my eyes, there was an amazing, clear, focussed view of pine boughs and needles and sunlight and little birds and sky and us sitting there, all One in a mysterious way.

Then I noticed, on this still, hot day, that the wind began to blow cool from the lake, until the pine needles whistled and sighed and I knew, somehow, that this was not just wind, but was the Presence, the Holy Wind, the Holy Spirit, the *Spiritus Sancti* moving through and around us. I became engulfed in this wind and in the Oneness of all and then heard in my mind a phrase I had been taught by the Inner Voice while writing *The Thomas Book*.

The Voice said, "I am in You: you are in Me." And as the voice repeated the phrase gently, over and over, I had an amazing sense of Oneness, of being within Oneness and Oneness being within me. I sensed that the phrase could be said either way: God saying, "I am in You: you are in Me," or me saying to God, "I am in You: You are in Me." God and Atman are One: "I and the Father are One."

There were no exclusions: everything was there, all the birds and grass and pine needles were there in the Oneness, and the voice kept repeating, "I am in you: you are in me," and I repeated back again, "I am in you: you are in me." I could feel God absolutely within me, and me somehow absolutely within God.

I quote from my journal, "Absolutely marvellous. It went on and on, lost in the sense of the Divine Words, 'I am in you: You are in Me,' and I knew God and myself and the world in Absolute Oneness and Peace -- all One but all absolutely distinct, each pine needle individual and clear and in God, shining forth God's Presence."

And I knew each blade of grass and each bird and Olive and Rachel sitting there and the people on the beach farther over beyond the trees and the Holy Wind surrounding all -- all One in the most glorious feeling of what it is to be One.

And I knew then what Yeshua meant when he said that all the hairs of our head are numbered and that God cares for the flowers and grass and birds and "will he not even more care for you?" I knew that Yeshua was not saying that God spends time counting hairs, but that God is within everything and that everything is within God, so that all these seemingly insignificant things are within the Consciousness of God and are actually a manifestation of that Divine Consciousness. How much more are we in God and God in us, if we can only bring ourselves to see without the barriers of our divisions?

I was absorbed in the sense of this amazing Oneness: one with God, with pine needles, with little birds and all the feathers on little birds, with the wind and the blades of grass and the people and even the rough bark on the tree trunks and the small bugs crawling on the bark. And I knew, without doubt, that the Inner Identity of All was actually God. It was as if I had always known at some level that this was the real nature of things, and I was now remembering who I really was and who the grass and the birds were, yet the perception had an amazing freshness, a tremendous newness to it.

I'm not sure how long this lasted. Then the Wind became calm, and the Voice within gradually faded without withdrawing, and I looked at the world, beginning to regain its distinctions and divisions, yet strangely peaceful now. It was as if I was coming back from a different world or a different way of being in the world which I had been privileged to share for a short time. For a short time I knew, without doubt, that God was in me and I was in God and God was in all things and we were all One.

Then the afternoon resumed, the flies buzzed, the birds hopped around in the trees and there we were, sitting on our blankets in the grass. But I had been allowed to get a glimpse of what the world really is beyond the divisions with which we live. And the experience has stayed with me, so that no matter what happens, I know that the divisions we think keep us from God and from each other are there only because we cannot yet see what the real nature of our relationships is, and we continue to do and think things which put up barriers to our true way of being in God's world.

Do I continue with the intensity of the Oneness all the time? No. We had to go back to our tent and cook and wash the dishes and return to the city to resume our usual life. The Vision was a gift, and has been repeated several times since in other ways. But it colours everything I do and think in the same way as your experiences in the Silence change your way of seeing and reacting to the world.

I still have to enter the Silence regularly to seek God's help and cleansing for error, and I still have to resolve conflict and misunderstanding, as we all do. But that is in the nature of our search for wholeness. In several places in the New Testament we are referred to as "those who are being perfected." We are not perfect, even though Yeshua encourages us to "Be perfect, even as your Father in Heaven is perfect" (Mat. 5:48).

Sometimes we are given a vision of what that perfect life can be, of the perfection and Oneness we can attain, and then we have to go back to work to try to develop that perfection in ourselves and to share that vision with others, and to work to establish the Kingdom of God on earth as in Heaven, because it is only together that we can achieve Oneness.

As you continue your practice of the Prayer of Silence, you will gradually realize that you are not the ego which identifies with the body and its possessions and position in society. You are the spiritual Ego, the I Am that is God. And, as you realize this, you will gradually develop within you what is called the Christ Consciousness, the awareness of oneness with God and with your fellow human beings.

As you Practice the Presence of God and become aware of how you are actually an expression, a manifestation of God, not theoretically, but deep within you, you will become the Light of God, the *Logos*, the Christ, the Anointed One of God – truly a Son or Daughter of God sharing in the Divine inheritance.

"I am in You. You are in Me." When it does not matter what order you say this in, whether you are in God or God is in you, or both, then you have come to the awareness of who you really are.

***

In this book I have tried to share with you where this Prayer of Silence can lead you, and how you can follow the path. And I have suggested something of the goal toward which you can work and some of the dangers along the way.

The next step -- and the next and the next -- comes only through regular practise. You continue to clear away enough of the errors and blockages from the inner Self, so that you perceive your Divine Nature more clearly, and so that you can hear within you the "still, small voice" which can guide you away from the dangers of condemnation, anger and hatred, to a life of forgiveness and love; so that you can develop a deep compassion for all people and for God's earth and all its creatures, and so that you can lead a life of service in the world. We do not seek to escape the world. We seek to enter more deeply into what the world really is, so that, ultimately, we know that we and the world and God are one.

Lightning Source UK Ltd.
Milton Keynes UK
UKHW011127200820
368549UK00006B/631